Big Food

Obesity is a global public health problem of crucial importance. Obesity rates remain high in high-income countries and are rapidly increasing in low- and middle-income countries. Concurrently, the global consumption of unhealthy products, such as soft drinks and processed foods, continues to rise. The ongoing expansion of multinational food and beverage companies, or 'Big Food', is a key factor behind these trends.

This collection provides critical insight into the global expansion of 'Big Food', including its incursion into low- and middle-income countries. It examines the changing dynamics of the global food supply, and discusses how low-income countries can alter the 'Big Food'-diet from the bottom-up. It examines a number of issues related to 'Big Food' marketing strategies, including the way in which they advertise to youths and the rural poor. These issues are discussed in terms of their public health implications, and their relation to public health activities, for example 'soda taxes', and the promotion of nutritionally-healthier products.

This book was originally published as a special issue of *Critical Public Health*.

Simon N. Williams is a Research Assistant Professor in the Department for Medical Social Sciences, Feinberg School of Medicine, Northwestern University, Chicago, Illinois, USA. His research focuses on how public health policy can help to regulate the rapid growth in the consumption of unhealthy products, including soft drinks and tobacco.

Marion Nestle is Paulette Goddard Professor in the Department of Nutrition, Food Studies, and Public Health at New York University, New York City, USA, and the author of three prize-winning books: *Food Politics: How the Food Industry Influences Nutrition and Health* (2007); *Safe Food: The Politics of Food Safety* (2010); and *What to Eat* (2007).

Big Food

Critical perspectives on the global growth
of the food and beverage industry

Edited by
Simon N. Williams and Marion Nestle

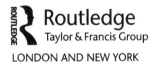

Routledge
Taylor & Francis Group

LONDON AND NEW YORK

First published 2016
by Routledge

2 Park Square, Milton Park, Abingdon, Oxfordshire OX14 4RN
711 Third Avenue, New York, NY 10017

Routledge is an imprint of the Taylor & Francis Group, an informa business

First issued in paperback 2017

British Library Cataloguing in Publication Data
A catalogue record for this book is available from the British Library

ISBN 13: 978-1-138-94594-4 (hbk)
ISBN 13: 978-1-138-30968-5 (pbk)

Typeset in Times New Roman
by RefineCatch Limited, Bungay, Suffolk

Publisher's Note
The publisher accepts responsibility for any inconsistencies that may have
arisen during the conversion of this book from journal articles to book chapters,
namely the possible inclusion of journal terminology.

Disclaimer
Every effort has been made to contact copyright holders for their permission to
reprint material in this book. The publishers would be grateful to hear from any
copyright holder who is not here acknowledged and will undertake to rectify
any errors or omissions in future editions of this book.

Contents

CONTENTS

Citation Information

The following chapters were originally published in *Critical Public Health*, volume 25, issue 3 (June 2015). When citing this material, please use the original page numbering for each article, as follows:

Editorial
'Big Food': taking a critical perspective on a global public health problem
Simon N. Williams and Marion Nestle
Critical Public Health, volume 25, issue 3 (June 2015) pp. 245–247

Chapter 1
The transitional dynamics of caloric ecosystems: changes in the food supply around the world
Sanjay Basu
Critical Public Health, volume 25, issue 3 (June 2015) pp. 248–264

Chapter 2
Big Food without big diets? Food regimes and Kenyan diets
K. O'Neill
Critical Public Health, volume 25, issue 3 (June 2015) pp. 265–279

Chapter 3
Density of outdoor food and beverage advertising around schools in Ulaanbaatar (Mongolia) and Manila (The Philippines) and implications for policy
Bridget Kelly, Lesley King, Batjargal Jamiyan, Nyamragchaa Chimedtseren, Bolorchimeg Bold, Victoria M. Medina, Sarah J. De los Reyes, Nichel V. Marquez, Anna Christine P. Rome, Ariane Margareth O. Cabanes, John Juliard Go, Tsogzolmaa Bayandorj, Marie Clem B. Carlos and Cherian Varghese
Critical Public Health, volume 25, issue 3 (June 2015) pp. 280–290

Chapter 4
Snack food advertising in stores around public schools in Guatemala
Violeta Chacon, Paola Letona, Eduardo Villamor and Joaquin Barnoya
Critical Public Health, volume 25, issue 3 (June 2015) pp. 291–298

Chapter 6

Comparison of food industry policies and commitments on marketing to children and product (re)formulation in Australia, New Zealand and Fiji
Gary Sacks, Melissa Mialon, Stefanie Vandevijvere, Helen Trevena, Wendy Snowdon, Michelle Crino and Boyd Swinburn
Critical Public Health, volume 25, issue 3 (June 2015) pp. 299–319

Chapter 7

Encouraging big food to do the right thing for children's health: a case study on using research to improve marketing of sugary cereals
Jennifer L. Harris, Megan E. LoDolce and Marlene B. Schwartz
Critical Public Health, volume 25, issue 3 (June 2015) pp. 320–332

Chapter 8

Big Soda's long shadow: news coverage of local proposals to tax sugar-sweetened beverages in Richmond, El Monte and Telluride
Laura Nixon, Pamela Mejia, Andrew Cheyne and Lori Dorfman
Critical Public Health, volume 25, issue 3 (June 2015) pp. 333–347

Chapter 9

'Big Food' and 'gamified' products: promotion, packaging, and the promise of fun
Charlene Elliott
Critical Public Health, volume 25, issue 3 (June 2015) pp. 348–360

Chapter 10

Food as pharma: marketing nutraceuticals to India's rural poor
Alice Street
Critical Public Health, volume 25, issue 3 (June 2015) pp. 361–372

The following chapter was originally published in *Critical Public Health*, volume 25, issue 4 (September 2015). When citing this material, please use the original page numbering for each article, as follows:

Chapter 5

The incursion of 'Big Food' in middle-income countries: a qualitative documentary case study analysis of the soft drinks industry in China and India
Simon N. Williams
Critical Public Health, volume 25, issue 4 (September 2015) pp. 455–473

For any permission-related enquiries please visit:
http://www.tandfonline.com/page/help/permissions

INTRODUCTION

'Big Food': taking a critical perspective on a global public health problem

Global increase in the consumption of low-nutrition products, such as soft drinks and processed foods, is associated with global increases in obesity and its associated diseases, most prominently type 2 diabetes (Basu, McKee, Galea, & Stuckler, 2013; Drewnowski & Popkin, 1997; Stuckler, McKee, Ebrahim, & Basu, 2012). The ongoing expansion of multinational food and beverage companies – 'Big Food' – is a key factor behind these increases in consumption (Stuckler & Nestle, 2012; Williams, in press). This special issue provides critical insight into the global marketing practices of Big Food, including a focus on their incursion into low-and middle-income countries (LMICs).

Despite all being focused on Big Food, the papers in this special issue are diverse in a couple of key respects. The studies focus on multiple countries: the US, Australia, New Zealand, Fiji, Mongolia, the Philippines, Guatemala, Kenya and India. They also employ multiple research methods such as quantitative analyses of food supply data-sets, qualitative interviews with key food policy stakeholders, ethnographic observations of the food marketing environment, geographic mapping of food advertisements and content analysis of documentation of food companies' public reports.

Taken together, these papers provide substantial evidence for the changing dynamics of the global food supply, including new insights into the 'nutrition transition' (Drewnowski & Popkin, 1997). This special issue deals particularly with issues related to the marketing strategies of Big Food, especially the ways in which companies advertise to youth and the rural poor. The papers demonstrate the importance of recent public health initiatives such as corporate promotion of nutritionally 'better for you' products and advocates' promotion of soda taxes.

The paper by Basu (2015) uses global food supply data to challenge the notion that changes in the food supply are a necessary consequence of economic development. He shows how such changes are more complex than a simple notion of 'Westernization' would have us assume. Instead, he argues we should consider the existence of multiple nutrition *transitions* and the extent to which they occur as the result of national policy choices as well as of global economic trends.

O'Neill's (2015) case study shows how Kenya, unlike many LMICs, has been slow to adopt the 'Big Food diet'. In that country, the availability of meats has remained constant and the availability of sugars and sweeteners has actually declined during what O'Neill refers to as the 'Corporate-Environmental food regime'. Although the Kenya case is an encouraging example of how multinational companies' expansion in LMICs can be checked by a state focus on national food self-sufficiency, it also warns us that most of the recent evidence suggests that 'the state's ability to manage food supplies is changing, and so are diets'.

Two studies in this issue examine the relationship between food and beverage advertising to school environments. In Mongolia and the Philippines (Kelly et al., 2015) and in Guatemala (Chacon, Letona, Villamor, & Barnoya, 2015), food advertising, in general, and child-oriented food advertising, in particular, were more frequent in areas nearer to schools. Chacon et al. (2015) also found that one-third of all snack food advertisements in stores within short walking distance of schools are child oriented.

Three of these articles focus on policies through which the adverse public health impacts of Big Food's expansion might be mitigated. Of the three, two (Harris, LoDolce, & Schwartz, 2015; Sacks et al., 2015) explore Big Food's voluntary commitments to (re)formulating healthier products and reducing child-directed marketing, whilst one (Nixon, Mejia, Cheyne, & Dorfman, 2015) examines media coverage of recent soda tax initiatives in the US. In their analysis of documents in Australia, New Zealand and Fiji, Sacks et al. (2015) observe that few prominent food companies have publically available policies related to the health effects of their products; those that do rarely address saturated fat, added sugar and overall energy density. Harris et al. (2015) evaluate the potential impact of a public health strategy to provide food companies with incentives to voluntarily improve child-targeted marketing practices. Their research found that after four years of incentives, companies had instituted some improvements in nutritional quality and marketing practices, although children's cereals were still less healthful than adult cereals. Finally, Nixon et al. (2015) offer a content analysis of news coverage of proposed soda taxes in three cities in California in the US. Their analysis provides insight into the ways in which Big Food fights such regulations in the mass media by, for example, using 'front groups' to make anti-tax arguments and by capitalizing on political tensions in the community.

This special issue also includes two commentaries. Elliott (2015) introduces 'gamification' as a new concept through which to analyse Big Food's marketing practices. She discusses how 'the promise of fun' is no longer exclusively associated with children's food. This focus on fun, she warns, may have the unintended consequence of encouraging people to eat more and 'sidestep issues of nutrition, calories, politics and health'. Finally, Street (2015) offers a critique of Big Food's marketing of 'nutraceuticals' to the rural poor in India. On a nutritional level, she questions the extent to which fortified foods should be promoted at the expense of natural and balanced diets. On an economic and cultural level, she questions the degree of saturation and impact such products can have in rural markets in LMICs.

It is now more than a decade since Marion Nestle wrote 'Food Politics' (Nestle, 2002, p. 1) to 'illuminate the extent to which the food industry determines what people eat and to generate wider discussion of the food industry's marketing methods and use of the political system'. This special issue will, we believe, stimulate even wider discussion by extending its scope to include new countries, concepts, methods and perspectives.

References

Basu, S. (2015). The transitional dynamics of caloric ecosystems: Changes in the food supply around the world. *Critical Public Health, 25*, 248–264.

Basu, S., McKee, M., Galea, G., & Stuckler, D. (2013). Relationship of soft drink consumption to global overweight, obesity, and diabetes: A cross-national analysis of 75 countries. *American Journal of Public Health, 103*, 2071–2077.

Chacon, V., Letona, P., Villamor, E., & Barnoya, J. (2015). Snack food advertising in stores around public schools in Guatemala. *Critical Public Health, 25*, 291–298.

Drewnowski, A., & Popkin, B. (1997). The nutrition transition: New trends in the global diet. *Nutrition Reviews, 55*, 31–43.

Elliott, C. (2015). 'Big Food' and 'gamified' products: Promotion, packaging, and the promise of fun. *Critical Public Health, 25*, 348–360.

Harris, J., LoDolce, M., & Schwartz, M. (2015). Encouraging big food to do the right thing for children's health: A case study on using research to improve. *Critical Public Health, 25*, 320–332.

Kelly, B., King, L., Jamiyan, B., Chimedtseren, N., Bold, B., Medina, V., ... Varghese, C. (2015). Density of outdoor food and beverage advertising around schools in Ulaanbaatar (Mongolia) and Manila (The Philippines) and implications for policy. *Critical Public Health, 25*, 280–290.

Nestle, M. (2013 [2002]). *Food politics: How the food industry influences nutrition and health.* Berkeley: University of California Press.

Nixon, L., Mejia, P., Cheyne, A., & Dorfman, L. (2015). Big Soda's long shadow: News coverage of local proposals to tax sugar-sweetened beverages in Richmond, El Monte and Telluride. *Critical Public Health, 25*, 333–347.

O'Neill, K. (2015). Big Food without big diets? Food regimes and Kenyan diets. *Critical Public Health, 25*, 265–279.

Sacks, G., Mialon, M., Vandevijvere, S., Trevana, H., Snowdon, W., Crino, M., & Swinburn, B. (2015). Comparison of food industry policies and commitments on marketing to children and product (re)formulation in Australia, New Zealand and Fiji. *Critical Public Health, 25*, 299–319.

Street, A. (2015). Food as pharma: Marketing nutraceuticals to India's rural poor. *Critical Public Health, 25*, 361–372.

Stuckler, D., McKee, M., Ebrahim, S., & Basu, S. (2012). Manufacturing epidemics: The role of global producers in increased consumption of unhealthy commodities including processed foods, alcohol, and tobacco. *PLoS Medicine, 9*, e1001235. doi:10.1371/journal.pmed.1001235

Stuckler, D., & Nestle, M. (2012). Big food, food systems, and global health. *PLoS Medicine, 9*, e1001242. doi:10.1371/journal.pmed.1001242

Williams, S. N. (in press). The incursion of 'Big Food' in middle-income countries: A qualitative documentary case study analysis of the soft drinks industry in China and India. *Critical Public Health, 25*. Published online, 2015, February 09.

Simon N. Williams
Department of Medical Social Sciences, Northwestern University, Chicago, USA.

Marion Nestle
Department of Nutrition, Food Studies, and Public Health, New York University, New York, USA.

The transitional dynamics of caloric ecosystems: changes in the food supply around the world

Sanjay Basu[a,b,c]

[a]Prevention Research Center, Centers for Health Policy, Primary Care and Outcomes Research, and Center on Poverty and Inequality, Stanford University, Stanford, CA, USA; [b]Department of Public Health and Policy, London School of Hygiene and Tropical Medicine, London, UK; [c]Stanford University School of Medicine, Stanford, CA, USA

Changes to the global food supply have been characterized by greater availability of edible oils, sweeteners, and meats – a profound 'nutrition transition' associated with rising obesity, type 2 diabetes, and cardiovascular disease. Through an analysis of three longitudinal databases of food supply, sales, and economics across the period 1961–2010, we observed that the change in global food supply has been characterized by a dramatic rise in pig meat consumption in China and poultry consumption in North America. These changes have not been experienced by all rapidly developing countries, and are not well explained by changes in income. The changes in food supply include divergence among otherwise similar neighboring countries, suggesting that the changes in food supply are not an inevitable result of economic development. Furthermore, we observed that the nutrition transition does not merely involve an adoption of 'Western' diets universally, but can also include an increase in the supply of edible oils that are uncommon in Western countries. Much of the increase in sales of sugar-sweetened beverages and packaged foods is attributable to a handful of multinational corporations, but typically from products distributed through domestic production systems rather than foreign importation. While North America and Latin America continued to have high sugar-sweetened beverage and packaged food sales in recent years, Eastern Europe and the Middle East have become emerging markets for these products. These findings suggest further study of natural experiments to identify which policies may mitigate nutritional risk factors for chronic disease in the context of economic development.

Introduction

Changes to the global food supply have been characterized by a dramatic shift in foods available for human consumption, particularly in low- and middle-income countries (Drewnowski & Popkin, 1997). The changes in food supply include greater availability of edible oils, caloric sweeteners, and animal source foods. These changes, collectively called the 'nutrition transition', have been statistically associated with rising obesity, type 2 diabetes, and cardiovascular disease worldwide (Basu, Stuckler, McKee, &

4

Galea, 2012; Basu, Yoffe, Hills, & Lustig, 2013; Popkin, 2001; Reddy & Yusuf, 1998; Yusuf, Reddy, Ôunpuu, & Anand, 2001).

Changes to the food supply have sparked increasing public concern about the nutrient quality of food availability around the world, the underlying factors such as trade agreements that are believed to be driving the nutrition transition in rapidly developing countries, and the role of 'Big Food' companies who manufacture and widely distribute processed foods associated with disease (Stuckler, McKee, Ebrahim, & Basu, 2012). Three key questions about the food supply are emerging in the setting of debates about how to best address the nutrition transition and Big Food companies. First, to what extent has the nutrition transition – described decades ago (Popkin, 1994) – continued, accelerated, or been mitigated among low- and middle-income countries in more recent years? The transition has been hypothesized to be accelerating in countries like India and China, where increasing consumption of Western-type diets is thought to be occurring in the context of rapid economic growth (Yang et al., 2010). Second, have all rapidly developing countries undergone the same transition or is the transition different among similar countries? If similar countries are undergoing different transitions – for example, if healthier foods are more available in one country than in neighboring countries undergoing similar social and economic changes – then differences in food supply may not be 'inevitable' consequences of economic development, but a product of specific policy choices. Third, what aspects of the transition are related to the actions of Big Food companies? Identifying which foods and companies are associated with increased unhealthy food supply may help identify future policy choices, reducing the impact of the nutrition transition on obesity, type 2 diabetes, and cardiovascular disease.

Here, we address these three questions using longitudinal data-sets describing food supply and food sales data from around the world. Because the nutrition transition has been particularly characterized by changes in the consumption of meats, edible oils, vegetables, and sugars, we particularly focused on these food groups in our analysis.

Methods

Data sources

We linked three large international longitudinal data-sets for our analysis. First, we used the UN Food and Agricultural Organization's (FAO) food balance sheets, which describe food supply among 216 countries from 1961 through 2007 in each of several standardized food groups (Food and Agricultural Organization, 2014). Second, we used the Euromonitor Passport Global Market Information (GMI) Database, which describes food sales per capita per year from 1997 through 2010 for each of several packaged or canned food products among 88 countries (Euromonitor International, 2013). Third, we used the World Bank World Development Indicators Database, which describes each country's gross domestic product per capita and dollars spent per year on food imports from 1961 through 2010 (World Bank, 2014).

Data analyses

We first analyzed trends in food supply per capita in the FAO Database for each of eight food categories within each country: cereals, sugar/sweeteners, meats, dairy/milk, fruits, vegetables, edible fats/oils, and fish/seafood. Food supply was expressed in kilocalories per capita per day, including only food directed to human consumption, excluding food waste, and food crops directed to products not for human consumption (e.g. animal feed).

5

We next conducted product-specific analyses of food sales in the GMI Database, focusing on beverages and packaged food products, with food sales expressed in exchange-rate-adjusted US dollars in purchasing power parity for comparability across countries, and in terms of net units sold per capita (US gallons for beverages, US tons for solid foods). We compared how food supply and food sales varied across regions and within regions, using World Bank classifications of countries into geographic blocks.

We finally regressed both food supply and food sales against GDP per capita and food import dollars to evaluate the correlations between income, food importation, supply and sales, and conducting fixed effects regressions to correct for time-invariant differences between countries. We specifically focused on GDP for this analysis because – while there are numerous changes associated with the nutrition transition (urbanization, agriculture changes, etc.), we specifically wished to determine whether GDP transitions routinely resulted in consistent nutrition transitions across countries, or if some countries underwent GDP increases without experiencing dramatic nutrition transitions. We report all regression results using population weights and robust standard errors clustered by the country. We conducted all analyses in Stata MP v. 12.1 (StataCorp, College Station, Texas).

Results

Trends in the nutrition transition

Changes in the food supply worldwide over the past five decades are illustrated in Figure 1. The greatest change in supply was the 204% rise in the supply of meat products – an increase from 109 kcals/capita/day in 1961 to 222 kcals/capita/day in 2007.

The large increase in meat supply was mostly in the form of pig meat and poultry meat, as shown in Figure 2. The increased meat supply in the form of pig meat occurred primarily in Southeast Asia, as shown in the figure. While pig meat supplies increased most substantially in China, the supplies simultaneously decreased in Western European and Central American countries. By contrast, the increase in poultry meat supply occurred in nearly all world regions, as shown in Figure 2. The increase in poultry meat was greatest in North America, where poultry meat consumption increased 316% from 64 kcals/capita/day in 1961 to 202 kcals/capita/day in 2007. As shown in the figure, increases in poultry meat supply also occurred to a lesser extent in Africa, Latin America, and Eastern Europe.

While smaller than the increase in meat supply, the vegetable supply also increased worldwide, as shown in Figure 3. The increase in vegetable supply was mostly in the form of corn and maize products. The increase in corn and maize products was greatest in North and West Africa, where a net increase of approximately 100 kcals/capita/day occurred between 1961 and 2007 in the context of large international aid shipments (i.e. not domestic production). Apart from these increases, further increases in vegetable supply per capita were also observed in Southeast Asia to a lesser extent.

In addition to changes in the meat and vegetable supply, a third notable transition worldwide was a change in edible oils, as shown in Figure 4. The increase in edible oils was mostly in the form of soybean and palm oils. As shown in the figure, the increase in soybean oil was observed mostly in Central Asia and Latin America, while palm oil supply increases were observed more in Southeast Asia and Latin America.

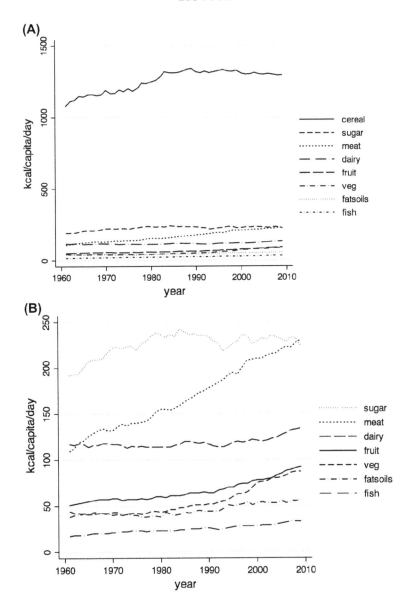

Figure 1. Changes to food supply worldwide (A) in all major food groups and (B) with cereals excluded to allow closer visualization of the rise in meat supply.

Variations among countries in the nutrition transition

We found that many low- and middle-income countries diverged from each other over the last five decades in terms of the changes in the food supply they experienced. The countries experiencing the largest changes in food supply within each of the major food groups are summarized in Table 1. As shown in the table, countries experiencing the largest changes in cereals were mostly African and Middle Eastern countries receiving large international aid shipments. However, variation in meat consumption appeared to

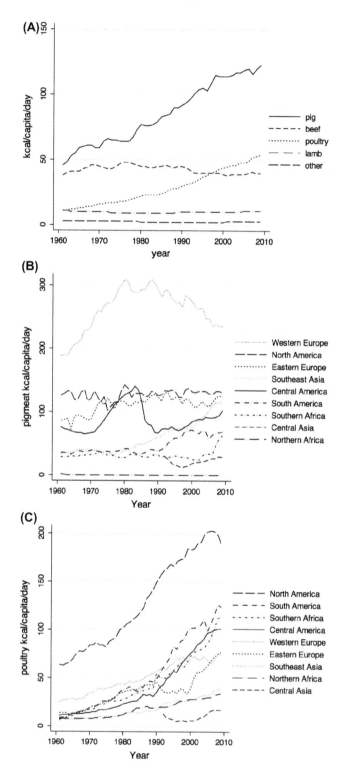

Figure 2. Rise in meat supply (A) worldwide; (B) specifically for pig meat, disaggregated by region; and (C) specifically for poultry meat, disaggregated by region.

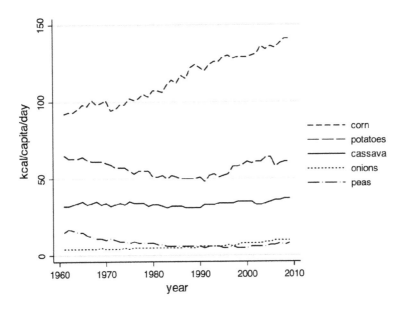

Figure 3. Vegetable supply changes worldwide.

be driven more by domestic production. As shown in the table and in Figure 5, China was unique among Asian countries in experiencing a large and sustained increase in meat supply per capita, mostly from domestic pig meat, while other Asian countries experienced a larger increase in sugar and sweetener supplies. For example, while China experienced a rise in meat consumption of over 350 kcals/capita/day from 1961 to 2007, South Korea and Thailand experienced smaller increases of 228 and 129 kcals/capita/day, respectively, even though all three countries experienced similar GDP per capita increases of around 160% during the period. China experienced a rise in the sugar supply of 62 kcals/capita/day, vs. 309 in South Korea and 264 in Thailand during the period 1961–2007, mostly in the form of imported sugar-containing products.

Different trends in food supply changes were observed in South Asia and Latin America. In South Asia, we observed that India, Pakistan, Bangladesh, and other countries of the region remained relatively stable in their consumption of all major food categories, as shown in Figure 5. In Latin America, countries also remained relatively stable in most food categories, except for a marked increase in sugar supply. The increase in sugar consumption was noted in all countries except Peru (Figure 5). Peru was also an exception from its neighbors for having maintained low dairy supplies and for having increased its fruit and vegetable supplies.

These differences in food supply trends were not explained by changes in GDP. As shown in Figure 6, GDP failed to explain a large portion of the variation in food supply among countries ($R^2 < 10\%$). Similarly, we observed that trends in food supply were not well explained by food importation. Food supply was more poorly explained by food importation than by GDP, as shown in Table 2. Looking further into the sources of food supply changes, we observed that most of the changes were associated with domestic food production, including domestic production of internationally franchised products, as explored in more detail in the next section.

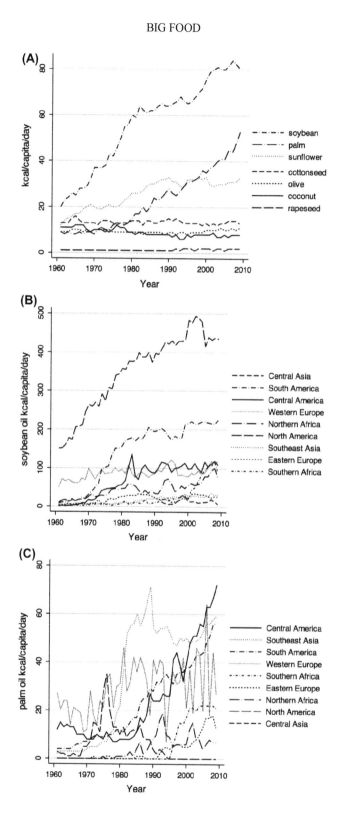

Figure 4. Edible oil supply changes (A) worldwide; (B) specifically for soybean oil, disaggregated by region; and (C) specifically for palm oil, disaggregated by region.

Table 1. Countries experiencing the largest changes in food supply in each food group, 1961–2007.

Country	Food group	Increase in kcals/capita/day, 1961–2007
	Cereals	
Palestine		1162
Burkina Faso		936
Algeria		728
Egypt		678
China		636
	Sugars	
South Korea		309
Thailand		264
Syria		261
Saudi Arabia		253
Palestine		247
	Meats	
China		388
Saint Lucia		358
Spain		352
Saint Vincent		317
Portugal		310
Samoa		307
	Dairy	
Albania		300
Romania		287
Greece		252
Dominica		214
Cape Verde		208
	Fruits	
Dominica		188
Sao Tome and Principe		182
Thailand		178
Cuba		154
United Arab Emirates		142
	Vegetables	
China		134
South Korea		113
Iran		110
Palestine		95
Malta		93
United Arab Emirates		90
	Fats and oils	
Vanuatu		176
Central African		107
Gabon		95
Benin		94
Samoa		92
	Fish	
Maldives		268
South Korea		76
Malaysia		66
Kiribati		65
Micronesia		65
	Total kcals	
Palestine		2240
Libya		1562
Colombia		1531
Algeria		1443
Dominica		1411
Iran		1363

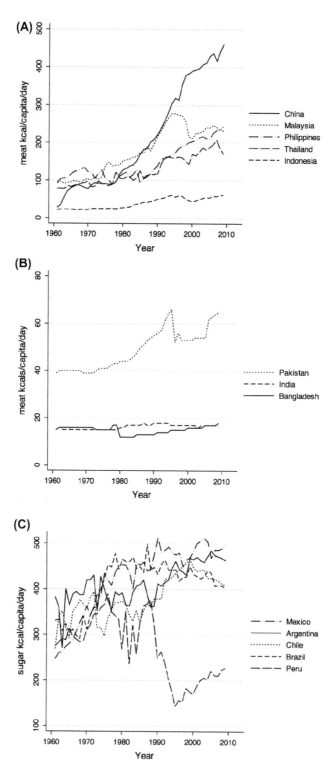

Figure 5. Intraregional supply changes: (A) in meat supply in Southeast Asia; (B) by contrast, relative stability in meat supply in South Asia despite economic growth in India; and (C) variations in sugar supply in Latin America.

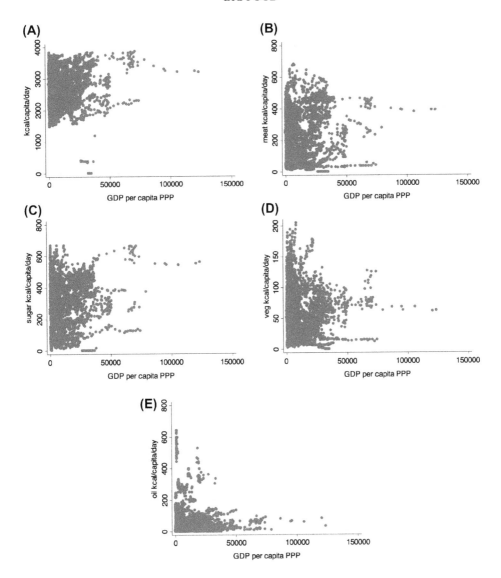

Figure 6. Variations in food supply vs. GDP: (A) total supply; (B) meat supply; (C) sugar supply; (D) vegetable supply; and (E) edible oil supply.

Trends in Big Food sales

Data from the food industry provide insights into how changes in food production and distribution are associated with overall changes in food supply. Data from the food industry are expressed in terms of changes in sales of products over time, clustered into two broad groups: beverage sales and packaged food sales.

Data from beverage sales reveal that beverages are an increasing source of sugar supply to populations worldwide. As shown in Figure 7, soda sales (sales of non-diet sugar-sweetened carbonated beverages) have increased from 9.4 to 11.2 gallons/capita/year worldwide from 1997 to 2010. But as shown in Table 3, soda sales have been highly divergent between countries and regions. While soda sales are widely known to

Table 2. GDP (per capita purchasing power parity in constant $US) and food imports ($US) vs. food supply (expressed in kcals/capita/day). $N = 216$ countries, 1961–2007.

Food group	vs. GDP	R^2	vs. food imports	R^2
Cereals	$-.0010^{**}$	.001	$-3.6e-10$	.000
Sugars	$.0022^{***}$	.033	$2.7e-9^{***}$	.015
Meats	$.0023^{***}$	.038	$3.1e-9^{***}$	.021
Dairy	$.0019^{***}$	.037	$9.7e-10^{***}$	.003
Fruits	$-.00030^{***}$	.003	$-1.7e-10$	.000
Vegetables	$.00025^{***}$	.008	$2.6e-10^{***}$	.003
Fats/oils	$-.00047^{***}$	.005	$-1.6e-11$	.000
Fish	$-.0000012$	.000	$2.9e-10^{***}$	.003
Total kcals	$.0077^{***}$	.034	$8.7e-9^{***}$	.011

$^*p < .05$; $^{**}p < .01$; $^{***}p < .001$.

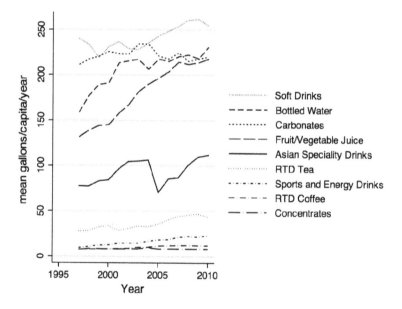

Figure 7. Soft drink sales worldwide.

be high in North America and Latin America, the greatest increase in sales over the studied period actually occurred in Eastern Europe and the Middle East, where many countries experienced over a 200 gallons/capita/year increase in sales from 1997 to 2010 (Table 2). Soda sales are also not universally high or increasing across Latin American countries, either. While soda sales were high in Mexico (averaging 521 gallons/capita/year) and Argentina (477 gallons/capita/year), for example, they remained substantially lower in Peru (48 gallons), Uruguay (44 gallons), Ecuador (56 gallons), and Colombia (55 gallons). Similarly, while soda sales were high in the United States (250 gallons/capita/year), they remained substantially lower in Canada (140 gallons).

Table 3. Countries experiencing the largest increase in carbonated non-diet soda and fruit/vegetable juice sales per capita per year, 1997–2010.

Country	Change in gallons/capita/year, 1997–2010
Soda	
Costa Rica	501
Greece	501
Kazakhstan	373
Ukraine	338
Georgia	314
Juice	
Germany	478
Russia	387
Serbia	373
Peru	323
Bulgaria	321

In parallel to the increase in soda sales, juices (from fruits and vegetables) increased in sales worldwide (Figure 7), with the largest increases observed again in Eastern Europe, the Middle East, and Latin America. While Peru maintained among the lowest levels of soda sales, it experienced among the highest increases in juice sales (323 gallons/capita/year). Similarly, Belarus decreased its soda sales by 290 gallons/capita/year from 1997 to 2010, while increasing its juice sales by 224 gallons/capita/year (see Table 3).

Data from processed food sales revealed similar increases in consumption in Eastern Europe and the Middle East. Most packaged food sales involved baked items (e.g. breads), dairy items (e.g. yogurts), confectionaries, and chilled processed foods (e.g. ready-to-eat meals). While packaged food sales were historically highest in Western Europe and North America, they increased in consumption most rapidly during the past decade in Eastern Europe, as shown in Figure 8.

As with data on overall food supply, the data on beverage sales and packaged food sales were not well explained by GDP or by food imports (Figure 9). At similar levels of GDP and of food importation, countries differed greatly in how much beverage and packaged food sales occurred, suggesting other factors may be critical for explaining international differences in sales trends.

Data from the food industry did reveal which companies were prominent in generating the majority of beverage and packaged food sales. These data reveal that the largest companies responsible for beverage and packaged food sales are multinational corporations who do not import most of their products to the affected countries, but often franchise local production. In terms of beverage sales, Table 4 reveals that the greatest sales worldwide are from Coca-Cola, followed by PepsiCo and Danone. We found little regional variation in which companies dominate beverage sales. In terms of packaged food sales, Table 4 also reveals that the greatest sales worldwide are from Nestle, followed by Kraft and Unilever. The distribution of market share among different regions is more varied in packaged food sales than in beverage sales, with the regional company Grupo Bimbo having a larger role in Latin America, but large North American multinationals otherwise dominating the landscape.

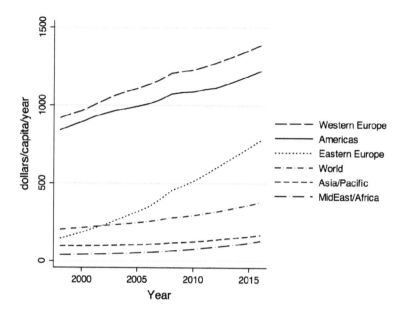

Figure 8. Packaged food sales worldwide.

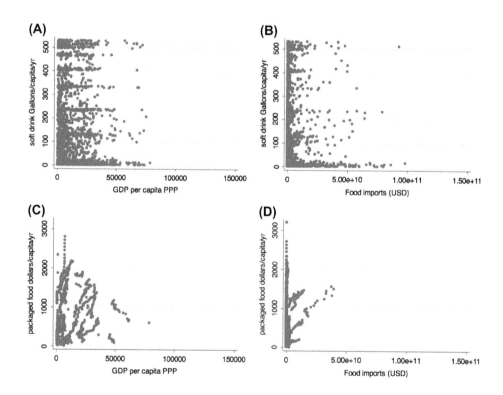

Figure 9. Variations on food sales vs. GDP and food imports. Soft drink sales vs. (A) GDP and (B) food imports. Processed foods sales vs. (A) GDP and (B) food imports.

Table 4. Top companies in terms of market share (total sales volume) worldwide in soft drinks and packaged foods, 1997–2010.

Company	Volume of sales	% of global market share
Soft drinks	(mn of liters)	
The Coca-Cola Co.	104,379.1	37.1
PepsiCo Inc.	48,662.0	17.3
Groupe Danone	21,838.5	7.8
Nestlé SA	18,741.9	6.7
Tingyi (Cayman Islands) Holdings Corp.	8020.9	2.9
Dr Pepper Snapple Group Inc.	7471.6	2.7
Suntory Holdings Ltd.	4884.1	1.7
Hangzhou Wahaha Group	3986.4	1.4
Aje Group	2870.1	1.0
Uni-President Enterprises Corp.	2635.2	.9
Packaged foods	($US millions)	
Nestlé SA	65,420.2	10.3
Kraft Foods Inc.	62,354.4	9.8
Unilever Group	39,366.6	6.2
PepsiCo Inc.	36,347.6	5.7
Mars Inc.	28,470.5	4.5
Groupe Danone	28,084.9	4.4
Kellogg Co.	16,059.0	2.5
General Mills Inc.	12,598.3	2.0
Ferrero Group	10,824.2	1.7
Grupo Bimbo SAB de CV	10,591.5	1.7

Discussion

Changes to the food supply across the world have been a source of increasing concern, as these food supply changes are thought to have a profound influence on the risk of chronic disease. Using data on food supply and food sales, we examined the extent to which the nutrition transition has been consistent or divergent between various regions and countries.

We observed several trends that contribute significant new knowledge to the existing literature. First, while it is well known that meat supply has been increasing (Popkin, 2006), our analysis clarified that much of this supply is concentrated in China (particularly in the form of pig meat) but is not necessarily inevitable in the context of economic development contrary to prior hypotheses (Speedy, 2003); India and other rapidly developing countries in Latin America, Africa, and other parts of Asia do not appear to be following China in their meat consumption. Meat consumption has also been driven by developed countries as well as low- and middle-income nations, for example, by the substantial rise in poultry consumption in North America. Second, our analysis revealed that the nutrition transition does not merely involve an adoption of 'Western' diets universally, but can also include an increase in the supply of edible oils that are uncommon in Western countries. The increased supply of foods uncommon in Western diets includes the increasing supply of palm oil in Southeast Asia and Latin America. The increasing supply of palm oil has been linked to cardiovascular disease (Chen, Seligman, Farquhar, & Goldhaber-Fiebert, 2011; Vega-Lopez, Ausman, Jalbert, Erkkila, & Lichtenstein, 2006). Third, our analysis revealed that large inter-regional differences exist between otherwise similar neighboring countries, even as entire regions undergo rapid economic development. For example, large inter-regional differences in Latin America reveal that the country of Peru has avoided the increases in sugar and dairy supply that some of its neighbors have experienced. This calls for further historical analysis into what factors may be contributing to Peru's divergence from other countries in the region, even when Peru has signed similar trade agreements and has experienced similar economic development as its neighbors (Organization of American States, 2014). Disaggregating the FAO data by total supply vs. imported supply alone would be important to regress against emerging data on trade liberalization by country, once such data are further standardized for analysis. Finally, we observed that while beverages and processed foods have generally increased in sales around the world, there is substantial variation in sales among countries, and the sales are not concentrated only in North America and Latin America, but also increasing in Eastern Europe and the Middle East, where less attention has been paid to their health implications.

Our findings provide several insights for future research endeavors. The divergence between otherwise similar countries provides a 'natural experiment' to investigate what domestic policies could be responsible for variations in food supply between countries. Understanding reasons for the divergence of Peru, for example, or the reasons why India and China diverge in even non-beef consumption (not religiously related meat consumption) could help determine which agriculture, trade, and nutrition policies are associated with food supply changes that may be responsible for improvements or decrements in human health. We found that large variations in food supply and sales cannot be explained by rising income or food importation alone. We also found that much of the increase in food supply and sales appears related to domestic production, including production from franchises of large multinational corporations. Hence, identifying how food supply and sales could be altered to improve public health will require further analysis of domestic variations in food policy, not just analyses of overall household income or international trade agreements. Such variations in domestic production policy could be added to international chronic disease policy monitoring databases that are in their early stages of data collection, such as the World Health Organization's chronic disease policy database (Stuckler & Basu, 2013; World Health Organization, 2014).

Our findings are limited, however, by caveats associated with the data used here. The findings are based on food supply and food sales, and hence are not as accurate proxies for actual food consumption as 24 hour dietary recalls or other direct dietary assessments, which are generally unavailable outside of North America and Europe. Food supply and food sales will tend to overestimate consumption where there is significant food wastages, as in the United States (Hall, Guo, Dore, & Chow, 2009). The findings also rely on data derived from formal food sales rather than informal bartering systems, and hence do not capture the complex dynamics of food supply in many lower-income countries. Finally, our between-country analyses do not account for complex within-country dynamics, which require more dedicated databases to study inequalities that are increasing in rapidly developing countries such as India.

As policy proposals to alter food supply continue to be proposed in an effort to address the global rise in chronic disease (Basu, Babiarz, et al., 2013; Basu et al., 2014), our analyses are a reminder that longitudinal trends in food supply have markedly diverged between nations, even among countries facing relatively similar socioeconomic changes. Further efforts are required to understand what explains this divergence even as we seek to address the health consequences of changing agricultural systems and changing diets worldwide.

References

Basu, S., Babiarz, K. S., Ebrahim, S., Vellakkal, S., Stuckler, D., & Goldhaber-Fiebert, J. D. (2013). Palm oil taxes and cardiovascular disease mortality in India: Economic-epidemiologic model. *British Medical Journal (Clinical Research Ed.), 347*, f6048.

Basu, S., Stuckler, D., McKee, M., & Galea, G. (2012). Nutritional determinants of worldwide diabetes: An econometric study of food markets and diabetes prevalence in 173 countries. *Public Health Nutrition, 1*(1), 1–8.

Basu, S., Vellakkal, S., Agrawal, S., Stuckler, D., Popkin, B., & Ebrahim, S. (2014). Averting obesity and type 2 diabetes in India through sugar-sweetened beverage taxation: An economic-epidemiologic modeling study. *PLoS Medicine, 11*, e1001582. doi:10.1371/journal.pmed.1001582

Basu, S., Yoffe, P., Hills, N., & Lustig, R. H. (2013). The relationship of sugar to population-level diabetes prevalence: An econometric analysis of repeated cross-sectional data. *PloS One, 8*, e57873. doi:10.1371/journal.pone.0057873

Chen, B. K., Seligman, B., Farquhar, J. W., & Goldhaber-Fiebert, J. D. (2011). Multi-country analysis of palm oil consumption and cardiovascular disease mortality for countries at different stages of economic development: 1980–1997. *Globalization and Health, 7*, 1–10.

Drewnowski, A., & Popkin, B. M. (1997). The nutrition transition: New trends in the global diet. *Nutrition Reviews, 55*, 31–43.

Euromonitor International. (2013). *Passport Global Market Information Database*. New York, NY: Author.

Food and Agricultural Organization. (2014). *FAOSTAT Database*. Rome: United Nations.

Hall, K. D., Guo, J., Dore, M., & Chow, C. C. (2009). The progressive increase of food waste in America and its environmental impact. *PLoS ONE, 4*, e7940. doi:10.1371/journal.pone.0007940

Organization of American States. (2014). *Foreign Trade Information System – Trade agreements in force*. Washington, DC: Author.

Popkin, B. M. (1994). The nutrition transition in low-income countries: An emerging crisis. *Nutrition Reviews, 52*, 285–298.

Popkin, B. M. (2001). The nutrition transition and obesity in the developing world. *The Journal of Nutrition, 131*, 871S–873S.

Popkin, B. M. (2006). Global nutrition dynamics: The world is shifting rapidly toward a diet linked with noncommunicable diseases. *The American Journal of Clinical Nutrition, 84*, 289–298.

Reddy, K. S., & Yusuf, S. (1998). Emerging epidemic of cardiovascular disease in developing countries. *Circulation, 97*, 596–601.

Speedy, A. W. (2003). Global production and consumption of animal source foods. *The Journal of Nutrition, 133*, 4048S–4053S.

Stuckler, D., & Basu, S. (2013). Malignant neglect: The failure to address the need to prevent premature non-communicable disease morbidity and mortality. *PLoS Medicine, 10*, e1001466. doi:10.1371/journal.pmed.1001466

Stuckler, D., McKee, M., Ebrahim, S., & Basu, S. (2012). Manufacturing epidemics: The role of global producers in increased consumption of unhealthy commodities including processed foods, alcohol, and tobacco. *PLoS Medicine, 9*, e1001235.

Vega-Lopez, S., Ausman, L. M., Jalbert, S. M., Erkkila, A. T., & Lichtenstein, A. H. (2006). Palm and partially hydrogenated soybean oils adversely alter lipoprotein profiles compared with soybean and canola oils in moderately hyperlipidemic subjects. *The American Journal of Clinical Nutrition, 84*, 54–62.

World Bank. (2014). *World Development Indicators*. Washington, DC: IBRD.

World Health Organization. (2014). *Nutrition, Obesity, and Physical Activity Database*. Geneva: Author.

Yang, W., Lu, J., Weng, J., Jia, W., Ji, L., Xiao, J., ... He, J. (2010). Prevalence of diabetes among men and women in China. *New England Journal of Medicine, 362*, 1090–1101. doi:10.1056/NEJMoa0908292

Yusuf, S., Reddy, S., Ounpuu, S., & Anand, S. (2001). Global burden of cardiovascular diseases: Part I: General considerations, the epidemiologic transition, risk factors, and impact of urbanization. *Circulation, 104*, 2746–2753.

Big Food without big diets? Food regimes and Kenyan diets

K. O'Neill

Department of Sociology, University of Toronto, Toronto, Canada

Path-breaking scholarship has described how corporate control of food production and distribution is implicated in the global emergence of diets heavy in fats, meats and sugars. The 'multinational food and beverage companies with huge and concentrated market power' can be thought of as Big Food. Big Food's presence in Kenya has expanded, and organizations have expressed concerns about the number of Kenyans who are obese. Despite these concerns, Kenya's dietary profile does not show a clear picture of high fats, meats and sugars. This suggests that the structural factors that shape the organization of Kenya's food supply need to be examined. By looking to the food regime approach, it is possible to understand how dietary patterns are a 'reconstitution of material culture', as trade arrangements shape diets in ways that make some foods seem traditional, while others appear to be new or exotic. By using the food regime approach, it is possible to understand how Kenya's position in international trade influences food production and consumption, as well as how the Kenyan state has played a role in mitigating the Big Food diet. In this respect, the policies and practices that organize Kenyan diets are reflective of global-historical arrangements, but are also particular to Kenya. I base my argument on ethnographic research conducted in 2010 and 2014 in urban and rural areas, interviews, FAOSTAT statistics, scholarship, government documents, agency reports, newspapers and relevant food websites.

Introduction

It once seemed counter-intuitive to expect increasing rates of heart disease, diabetes and obesity in countries characterized by malnourishment. Thanks to path-breaking scholarship, we are aware that changing diets in different parts of the world are linked to these health outcomes (Drewnowski & Popkin, 1997; Patel, 2007; Popkin, 1993, 2006). In Kenya, concerns about diabetes and obesity are regularly discussed in newspapers (Muraya, 2014; Ndemwa, 2013; Ngwiri, 2014), which relates to research examining Kenyans' new dietary leanings (Raschke & Cheema, 2008; Steyn, Nel, Parker, Ayah, & Mbithe, 2012; Vorster, Kruger, & Margetts, 2011).

Dietary changes, specifically, diets heavy in fats, meats and sugars, have emerged in tandem with the growth of corporate control over food production and distribution (Hawkes, 2006; Nestle, 2002/2013; Patel, 2007; Popkin, 1993; Weis, 2007). The 'multinational food and beverage companies with huge and concentrated market power'

(Stuckler & Nestle, 2012, p. 1) can be described as Big Food. The global value of food trade has grown tremendously in recent decades, but '[v]irtually all growth in Big Food's sales occurs in developing countries' (Stuckler & Nestle, 2012, p. 1). Big Food is not just involved in selling products in newly open markets, but acting politically in order to ensure that it can access markets (Nestle, 2002/2013; Patel, 2007; Weis, 2007). These actions involve lobbying international organizations to access closed markets, state agencies to pass favourable regulations, and nutritional and health experts to promote some food claims over others (Clapp & Fuchs, 2009; Nestle, 2002/2013; Patel, 2007; Weis, 2007).

Despite concerns about dietary quality and autonomy amidst the growth of Big Food, there is no strong evidence that the Big Food diet has been taken up by Kenyans. This flies in the face of research on global dietary changes, as well as reported health concerns. The goal of this article is to identify some of the links between the local–national and the international political economy of food to better understand why the Big Food diet is not widespread in Kenya. I argue that the state has played a major role in mitigating diets, and this role becomes clearer if we use the food regime approach to understand how Kenya's position in international trade influences food production and consumption. I base my argument on six months of ethnographic research conducted in 2010 and 2014 in urban and rural areas, including almost daily visits to food retailing outlets such as wet markets, supermarkets, corner stores, hyper markets, fast-food outlets, restaurants and roadside vendors. I triangulated ethnographic observations with more than 70 interviews with farmers, national and county government officials, and NGO representatives, FAOSTAT food supply, production, and trade statistics, scholarship, government documents, agency reports, newspapers, and relevant food websites.

Big Food and Kenya's foodscape

Research has pointed to several factors that predict shifts to the Big Food diet such as urbanization, the growth of the middle class, less physically taxing work demands and the rise of food capitals (De Vogli, Kouvonen, & Gimeno 2011; Drewnowski & Popkin, 1997; Hawkes, 2005, 2006; Patel, 2007; Popkin, 1993, 2006; Raschke & Cheema, 2008). Kenya has been described as having the leading economy in East Africa (Kabukuru, 2009, p. 64), and its urban middle class has emerged as new buyers of goods ranging from housing to cosmetics (Daily Nation, 2014a, 2014b; Maina, 2014; Neven, Reardon, Chege, & Wang, 2006). It is important to be cautious of overgeneralizing the disposable income that the middle class has though (Ravallion, 2009). The nutritional and economic pressures many Kenyans face are quite serious, and roughly 25% of the population is malnourished (FAO, 2014).

Kenya's 'supermarket revolution' began in the late 1990s, and supermarkets' market share is growing (Neven & Reardon, 2004, p. 669; Neven et al., 2006; Neven, Odera, Reardon, & Wang, 2009). Supermarkets are able to provide a wider range of processed food items, sometimes at a lower price, and often in a variety of sizes and price points. Flyers, loyalty programs and sales encourage shopping, with some stores providing a 'lifestyle' experience by offering shoes, clothing, furniture, electronics and home décor in addition to food. Consumers of different classes now shop in the same food retail outlets for different items (Neven & Reardon, 2004; Neven et al., 2006). With deli counters providing hot meat and cheese pies for around $2, as well as customary dishes of ugali and sukuma wiki, it seems that supermarkets are savvy to what their customers want.

Supermarkets are not the only retailers implicated in dietary changes; fast-food restaurants and food-brand competitors are also involved. Domestic and regional fast-food restaurants emulate Big Food strategies by using aggressive marketing to encourage brand recognition and consumption, and by coordinating the production of consistent, ready-to-eat foods (Gereffi & Christian, 2010; Matejowsky, 2009; Ritzer, 2006). In Kenya, Steers, Galito's, Chicken Inn, Pizza Inn, Creamy Inn, Kentucky Fried Chicken and Subway (amongst others) are opening more outlets to serve a wider client base. Many stores offer daily specials, family meal packages and delivery options (Creamy Inn, 2011; Steers, 2014a). These restaurants engage in a fight over brand loyalty as they offer signature dishes such as boerewors pizza or peri-peri and cheese chicken burgers (Pizza Inn, 2013; Steers, 2014b). Some of the restaurants have the additional 'brand value' of being described by customers as African success stories (Galito's, 2011).

The competition for brand loyalty is evident in television advertisements, posters and newspaper stories. Pepsi and Coca-Cola's fight for market share has been featured in national newspapers (David, 2014; Gikunju, 2013). Their sponsorship of projects is likely a part of this fight. For instance, Coca-Cola supplied more than a million dollars in a grant programme in partnership with the Ministry of Devolution and Planning (Otieno, 2013). This programme supplies small fridges, umbrellas and crates of soda to women and youth, presenting them with business opportunities. Understandably, the appearance of Big Food can be viewed positively by government agencies interested in attracting investment and providing employment (Hawkes, 2005).

Based on this picture, it would seem plausible to expect that major dietary changes are underway in Kenya. Moreover, various organizations have expressed concern about the growing number of Kenyans who are overweight and obese, seemingly speaking to the presence of a dietary shift (Ndemwa, 2013; Wanja, 2010; World Health Organization [WHO], 2011). Yet, the dietary profiles for Kenya do not reflect such an obvious change, suggesting that the structural factors that shape the way Kenya's food supply is organized need to be examined.

The Big Food diet: fats, meats and sugars in Kenya

The pattern of dietary shifts in low- and middle-income countries from grains, legumes and fibres to fats, meats and sugars is often referred to as 'the nutrition transition' (Drewnowski & Popkin, 1997; Popkin, 1993, 1994; WHO, 2011). The increased consumption of vegetable fats as opposed to animal fats 'is a key to the early phase' of dietary changes (Hawkes, 2010, p. 35). But it is only recently that research is looking into Kenyan diets (Mendez, Monteiro, & Popkin, 2005; Raschke & Cheema, 2008; Steyn et al., 2012; Vorster et al., 2011), and more work is needed to explore if and how Big Food is involved.

In terms of the availability of fats, meats and sugars, it is clear that vegetable oil or like products rose sharply in Kenya in the late 1970s (Figure 1). The second spike in vegetable oils takes place in the early 1990s; however, Kenya's dietary profile does not reflect similar increases in the availability of meats and sugars (Figures 2 and 3). If anything, the amount of beef available for consumption has decreased until recently

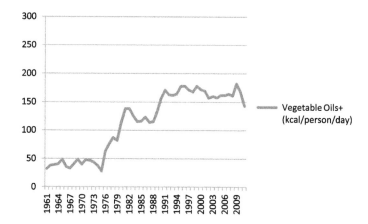

Figure 1. The amount of vegetable oils available for consumption in Kenya, 1961–2011. Source: FAOSTAT (2014a).

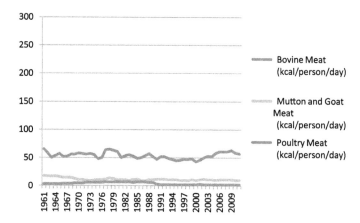

Figure 2. The amount of meat available for consumption in Kenya, 1961–2011. Source: FAOSTAT (2014a).

(2000), mutton and goat have stayed fairly stable since the early 1970s, and chicken has declined since the early 1990s.

In contrast to the amount of fats and meats available for consumption, sugars and sweeteners experienced a major jump from the early 1970s to the late 1980s, only to drop back to 1960s quantities by the late 1990s (Figure 4). There has been a rise in sugar and sweetener availability since the late 1990s, though levels are still lower than what they were in the 1980s. Since 2003, there has been an increase in sugar cane availability, but not enough to make up for the loss of refined sugar availability which comprises 95–99% of the sugars and sweeteners available in any given year (Figure 5).

Taking fats, meats and sugars together, it is possible to look at the FAOSTAT profiles and surmise that diets are in the early stages of change. By drawing on the food regime approach though, it is possible to have a more nuanced view of some of the structural conditions that are important to the manifestation of Big Food diets.

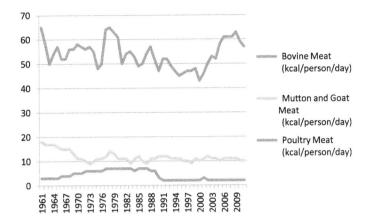

Figure 3. A closer examination of the amount of meat available for consumption in Kenya, 1961–2011.
Source: FAOSTAT (2014a).

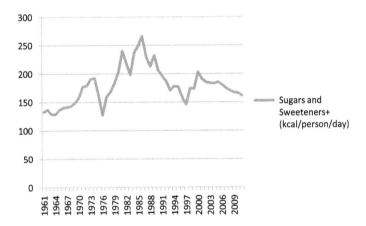

Figure 4. The amount of sugars and sweeteners available for consumption in Kenya, 1961–2011.
Source: FAOSTAT (2014a).

Linking dietary shifts to trade arrangements: the food regime approach

The food regime approach can be used to examine the organization of Kenya's food supply and impacts to Kenya's foodscape. Food regimes refer to relatively stable periods in the international political economy of food, characterized by specific forms of capital accumulation that manifest in geographical and classed patterns of food production and distribution (Friedmann, 1992, 1999, 2005; Friedmann & McMichael, 1989; McMichael, 2005, 2009). This approach was pioneered by Friedmann and McMichael in 1989 and is useful to contextualize and interpret global trends in food consumption by 'historici[zing] the global food system: problematizing linear representations of agricultural modernization' (McMichael, 2009, p. 140). The food regime approach points us towards understanding how dietary patterns are a 'reconstitution of material culture' (McMichael, 2005, p. 288), as trade arrangements are reflected in diets in ways that make some foods seem traditional, while others appear to be new or exotic

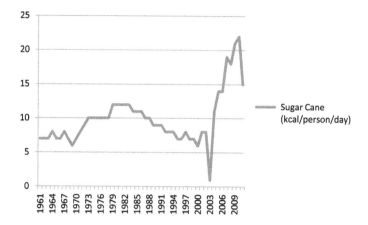

Figure 5. The amount of sugar cane available for consumption in Kenya, 1961–2011.
Source: FAOSTAT (2014a).

(Friedmann, 1992, 1999, 2005). In this way, the food regime approach provides an analytical lens to interpret how Big Food products appear in a region and become a feature of diets.

We can make sense of the Big Food diet with reference to the rise of fats, meats and sugars during two food regimes, namely the Mercantile-Industrial food regime (1950s–1970s) and the Corporate-Environmental food regime (1980s-present). In the Mercantile-Industrial food regime, the conditions were set for the Big Food diet to arise mainly in wealthy countries, while in the Corporate-Environmental food regime the presence of fats, meats and sugars are facilitated in low- and middle-income countries.

In the Mercantile-Industrial food regime, technological advancements in the production of vegetable fats led to greater quantities and varieties of cooking fats, spreads and oils (Drewnowski & Popkin, 1997). As countries engaged in oil crop subsidization and export, vegetable fats became more globally available and affordable (Drewnowski & Popkin, 1997; Friedmann, 1992). Scientific innovations also led to new sweeteners, which stabilized supplies when sugar prices rose, and provided a sweet maize-based alternative to sugar (Friedmann, 1992). Moreover, feedstuffs for livestock were created with maize and soy, making concentrated animal feedlots viable (Friedmann, 1992; Weis, 2007). Agribusinesses linked grains to meat production, and '... elaborated transnational linkages between national farm sectors, which were subdivided into a series of specialised agricultures linked by global supply chains' (McMichael, 2009, p. 141). Altogether, the national subsidizing of crops, intensification of industrialized agriculture and rise of global supply chains made fats, meats and sugars cheaper and widely available to consumers with disposable incomes (Friedmann, 1992, 2005; Weis, 2007).

At the same time, the rise of this diet was limited because '... international markets operated like canal locks between national markets ... Countries only traded surpluses and shortages on the international market in the quantities required ...' (Daviron, 2008, pp. 59–60). This pattern of food trade changed with market liberalization in the 1980s. Countries that entered into structural adjustment loans were encouraged by lenders to develop 'non-traditional' exports such as horticulture and aquaculture while opening their borders to food imports (Friedmann, 2005). The resulting pattern of trade is of 'a politically constructed division of agricultural labour between Northern staple grains traded for Southern high-value products (meats, fruits and vegetables)' (McMichael, 2009, p. 148). These geopolitical food flows can be characterized in terms of basic and luxury foods (Otero, Pechlaner, & Gürcan, 2013), but it is important to qualify how food production is consequently organized. The basic foods that are imported can be used towards intensifying the domestic production of fats, meats and sugars as well as export production (Delgado, 2003; Friel et al., 2013; Hawkes, 2010; Thow & Hawkes, 2009). This means that the import of basic foods can manifest in Big Food diets.

Though the food regime approach can be used to interpret the rise of the Big Food diet, it 'makes no claim to comprehensive treatment of different agricultures across the world' (McMichael, 2009, p. 140). In this respect, Daviron (2008) has examined the marginalization of African countries in the international political economy of food. He describes global food trade from the 1970s onwards as characterized by 'differentiation of trading conditions, with price differentiation according to destination, specific credit conditions, the development of barter operations, etc.' (Daviron, 2008, p. 74). Questions about differentiation can be addressed by examining 'how and whether their [states'] internal sociopolitical dynamics ... alter dominant trends' (Pechlaner & Otero, 2010, p. 204). Following this line of analysis, Otero et al. (2013) and Pechlaner and Otero (2010) have proposed that the food regime operating from the 1980s onward should be referred to as the Neoliberal food regime, because the title 'Neoliberal' versus 'Corporate-Environmental' serves as a reminder that states are key actors in creating and implementing trade arrangements.

In order to understand the dietary changes taking place in a country then, it is important not only to look at the presence of Big Food itself, but how the supply of fats, oils and sugar is organized. The organization of supply impacts how foods are available and accessible. Kenya's history of national agri-food policies during the Mercantile-Industrial and Neoliberal periods in the international political economy of food reveals specific impacts for fats, meats and sugars, and for diets.

The Mercantile-Industrial food regime

While the policies and practices that organize Kenyan diets are reflective of global-historical arrangements, they are also particular to Kenya. The Mercantile-Industrial food regime overlaps the last few years of Kenya's colonization and independence (1963). Despite differences in governance, this period is characterized by the state's regulation of food production and trade.

By orienting farmers to the production of export crops such as pyrethrum, coffee and tea, the Kenyan government expected to improve its GDP and invest in industry (Government of Kenya, 1965; Swynnerton, 1954). With independence (1963), the government purchased under-used and abandoned European settler plots using loans and distributed them to landless Kenyans. For example, the Million Acre strategy involved the purchase of European lands using funds borrowed from Britain, Germany and the World Bank (Hebinck, 1990; Maxon, 1992; Winter-Nelson, 1995). This plan built on a prior strategy to incent Kenyans towards agricultural production vis-à-vis individual, registered tenure (Cowen & Shenton, 1996; Leys, 1975; Maxon, 1992; Ochieng', 1992; Swynnerton, 1954; Winter-Nelson, 1995). The Kenyatta government (1964–1978) made yield estimates based on farm sizes and features and looked to agricultural production as collateral for Kenyans' new lands (Hebinck, 1990; Leys, 1975; Ochieng', 1992; Winter-Nelson, 1995).

The state also invested in technology, provided maize seeds to farmers at little to no cost and subsidized fertilizer and pesticides (Hebinck, 1990). The government encouraged farmers to dairy and plant maize so that farmers had a reliable supply of food until they successfully transitioned into the cash economy (Ministry of Finance and Economic Planning, 1971). Food producers typically relied on maize and milk for more than 60% of their total consumption (Ministry of Finance and Economic Planning, 1971, p. 55), while smallholders outside of settlement schemes were 'reliant on his staple foods, livestock and milk, not only as sources of most of his food, but also as the main sources of his farm income' (Casley & Marchant, 1979, p. 24).

In an attempt to reduce import costs, the government invested in large-scale sugar milling factories, and its shareholdings ranged from 71 to 98.5% (Jabara, 1985, p. 613). Throughout the 1970s, the availability of sugar cane rose in rough correspondence to increased producer prices (Jabara, 1985). The state also supported vegetable oil production. For instance, Unilever acquired a 50% share of East Africa Industries in 1953, and the colonial government agreed to protect it from competition providing it made vegetable oil available at 'favourable' prices (in Swainson, 1980, p. 144). When East Africa Industries faced difficulty sourcing cotton seed from Uganda, it switched to the cheaper palm, sourcing supplies from its plantations in Zaire and Malaysia (Dinham & Hines, 1984; Jabara, 1985).

Though the Mercantile-Industrial food regime made cheap oils, meat and sugar available to consumers in wealthy countries, measures taken by the Kenyan government worked to ensure that citizens had supplies of domestically processed and regulated vegetable oil and sugar, along with maize and milk. Starting in the 1970s though,

> ... a series of "shocks" – oil price and dollar fluctuations, debt and financial crisis, the rise of NICs – ... [shook] ... the nation-centred growth model. Since the mid-1970s, the OECD countries ... [began] ... to reform their economies in response to these shocks. Privatization, deregulation and the opening of national markets have been the basic ingredients in the liberal regime that has been adopted by these countries. (Daviron, 2008, p. 64)

By 1977, Kenya's total loans comprised 11.2% of GDP (Hebinck, 1990, p. 74). With changing ideas about domestically regulating food (Daviron, 2008; Friedmann, 2005) and Kenya's rising debt to GDP ratio, international lenders demanded changes in Kenya's economic structuring.

The Neoliberal food regime

The change from the Mercantile-Industrial regime to the Neoliberal regime is marked by economic restructuring. Kenya's structural adjustment loan required the phasing out of government intervention in food and agriculture. Loan conditions stipulated that parastatals could continue to ensure food reserves, but could not set prices, import quotas, or regulate domestic markets (Nyangito, Nzuma, Ommeh, & Mbithi, 2006; Swamy, 1994). Despite these conditions, the Moi government (1978–2002) maintained import restrictions on commodities that competed with domestic production (Nyangito et al., 2006; Swamy, 1994).

Kenya's economy became officially 'open' or liberalized in 1993 when The World Bank made it clear that funds would not be released as planned unless the government submitted to conditions (Nyangito et al., 2006; Odame, Musyoka, & Kere, 2009; Swamy, 1994). Even though the Kenyan government was required to reduce its involvement in agriculture and food, President Kibaki (2002–2013) put a Price Control Act into place, allowing it to fix prices of essential commodities including maize, wheat and rice (as well as their flours), cooking fats, and sugar (Government of Kenya, 2009). Parastatals continue to exercise some discretion over food supply and make changes in import tariff rates, ban exports and use treasury funds for food purchases (Ariga & Jayne, 2010).

Since the late 1980s, the amount of maize available for consumption has declined, and the amounts of rice and wheat available for consumption have increased in rough correspondence (Figures 6 and 7). Urban, middle-class consumers are frequently enjoying bread and wheat-based convenience foods, as well as rice (Muyanga, Jayne, Argwings-Kodhek, & Ariga, 2005). Although production of maize, rice and wheat has generally risen (FAOSTAT, 2014b), Kenya imports these cereals. Maize primarily comes from the East African region, wheat from the Ukraine, Pakistan, Russia and Argentina, and rice from Pakistan and Vietnam (Andae, 2014; FAOSTAT, 2014c).

Kenya's trade with these countries reflects its status as a member of the World Trade Organization, and it became a member in 1995 (Nyangito et al., 2006). For members of the WTO, trade must take place via the most-favoured-nation clause in order to prevent selective trade advantages (WTO, 2013). Yet regional trade agreements allow countries to create advantages, sometimes with preferential clauses (Friel et al., 2013; WTO, 2013). Kenya is a member of a common market agreement for Eastern and Southern Africa known as COMESA. Kenya's domestic sugar industry is protected by the limits on the amount of sugar to be imported through COMESA, and additional taxes and licensing are applied to non-COMESA imports (Apollo, 2014; Gibendi, 2014a). Kenya's sugar protections are set to expire in 2015, and the parastatal Kenya Sugar Board is in the process of being dismantled (Gibendi, 2014a, 2014b), which suggests that cheaper sugar will compete with domestic products.

Confectionery manufacturers like Lindt point to increasing interest in the Kenyan market despite fluctuations in sugar supplies (Maina, 2012; Okeyo, 2012). As one journalist stated, 'Annual per capita consumption of Coca-Cola … in Kenya is 39 servings. In more developed countries like Mexico, which consumes more Coca-Cola than any other country, it runs 665 servings per year. One does not need an MBA to see the possibilities'

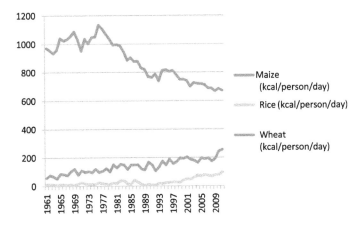

Figure 6. The amount of maize, rice and wheat available for consumption in Kenya, 1961–2011. Source: FAOSTAT (2014a).

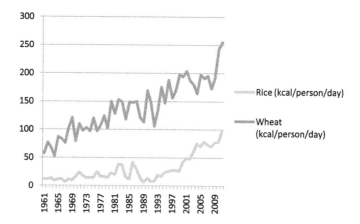

Figure 7. A closer examination of the amount of rice and wheat available for consumption in Kenya, 1961–2011.
Source: FAOSTAT (2014a).

(Stanford, 2010). Vendors bring sugary offerings such as $0.06 lollipops and $0.40 sodas to potential customers who are waiting for buses, stopped in traffic, or seated in parks. In rural and urban areas, bakeries serve small loaves of frosted cakes and cupcakes ranging from $0.35 to a little over a dollar. There is a range of affordability that tends to vary inversely with portion size, and cheaper sugar could make greater quantities of confectionary available to Kenyans.

Like with sugars, meat availability does not conform to Big Food diets. However, Kenchic established its own broiler factory farm in the early 1980s, producing 20,000 chicks per week (Kenchic, 2012). These chickens supply Kenchic Inn restaurants, competitors such as Kentucky Fried Chicken and Steers (Kenchic, 2012), and some supermarkets' freezers. An Egyptian agribusiness firm has plans to compete with Kenchic's factory farming strategies (Gibendi, 2013). The firm aims to make Kenya fully self-sufficient in chicken by 2019 and also aims to export (Gibendi, 2013). The need to adopt industrial rearing standards for export is not widespread; export volumes make up 1% of Kenya's meat production (Farmer & Mbwika, 2012).

Rather than adopt the factory farming model, many of the farmers I spoke with produced their own feed for some or all of their animals' needs because of the expense of feedstuffs. The farmers who used zero-grazing methods explained that they confined animals due to a shortage of farmhands or grazing land. Farmers consider how well-suited animals are to their locales in addition to other characteristics, such as milk production or meat characteristics. These factors influence why about three-quarters of Kenya's chicken are indigenous and free range (Gibendi, 2013). Furthermore, the bulk of Kenya's livestock are supplied by its pastoralists, and the 20–25% of livestock imported from neighbouring African countries can be expensive (Farmer & Mbwika, 2012, p. 37).

The Kenya Meat Commission and private abattoirs supply meat to restaurants and supermarkets (Farmer & Mbwika, 2012; KMC, 2014), but households will butcher a chicken for dinner or a goat for a celebratory feast. Meat is not an essential feature of most meals and when present, the portions tend to be modest in comparison with

American servings. In urban centres and likely rural as well, 'the middle class accounts for the large majority of meat consumers ...' (Farmer & Mbwika, 2012, p. 6).

In contrast, vegetable oils do conform to the Big Food diet. In Figure 1, it can be seen that the second spike in vegetable oils coincides with Kenya's structural reforms. By 2005, vegetable oil imports into Kenya were second in importance to petroleum (EPZA, 2005, p. 1). Vegetable fats are amongst the top ten ingredients commonly consumed by Kenyan women (Steyn et al., 2012), and advertisements for these products tend to emphasize their health benefits. For instance, Blue Band margarine is described as containing the daily amounts of essential fats and vitamins needed for children's healthy development (Unilever, 2014), and Bidco vegetable fats are described as potentially having cancer-fighting properties (2014). Some of the women I spoke with described bread and margarine as a healthy breakfast or snack they could prepare in a hurry for household members. Oils and small packages of margarine usually do not need to be refrigerated, so using oils when preparing foods can be a way of enhancing flavours and integrating health claims, with varied significance for consumers of different genders and classes (Steyn et al., 2012).

Conclusion

The growing presence of food capitals in Kenya has not resulted in the general adoption of the Big Food diet. Instead, the way that food production has been organized has had an impact on the kinds of foods available to be eaten. The Kenyan state has been influential in organizing production, and its focus on national food self-sufficiency has regularly characterized agri-food practices. However, the state's ability to manage food supplies is changing, and so are diets.

Some Kenyans are replacing maize with wheat and rice-based foods. It is possible that greater sugar and meat consumption will follow, particularly as domestic protections expire, or if factory farming gains a foothold. This article cannot predict the future, but has illustrated some of the factors that support the emergence of Big Food diets. Nevertheless, there is an obvious shortfall: more research is needed to understand how Kenyans of varying backgrounds engage with and want to engage with diverse food options.

Acknowledgements

I am grateful for Harriet Friedmann's feedback on prototypes, and Daniel Silver's, Erik Schneiderhan's and Salina Abji's support on the later version. I sincerely thank two anonymous reviewers for their perceptive comments and constructive suggestions.

Funding

I gratefully acknowledge the financial support of the Canadian International Development Agency through the Association of Universities and Colleges of Canada's Students for Development Program, the Muriel D. Bissell Award and the University of Toronto School of Graduate Studies Travel Grant.

References

Andae, G. (2014). Kenya plans maize import in May as shortage looms. *Daily Nation*. Retrieved from http://www.businessdailyafrica.com/Kenya-plans-maize-import-in-May/-/539546/2143598/-/1ke7cgz/-/index.html

Apollo, S. (2014). Sugarcane farmers issue bitter ultimatum. *Daily Nation*. Retrieved from http://www.nation.co.ke/business/Cane-farmers-to-boycott-over-illegal-sugars-imports/-/996/2252882/-/o6b8o/-/index.html

Ariga, J., & Jayne, T. (2010). Maize trade and marketing policy interventions in Kenya. In A. Sarris & J. Morrison (Eds.), *Food security in Africa: Market and trade policy for staple foods in eastern and southern Africa* (pp. 221–251). Cheltenham: Edward Elgar.

Bidco. 2014. *Vegetable cooking fats*. Retrieved from http://www.bidco-oil.com/bidco-products/vegetable-cooking-fats

Casley, D. J., & Marchant, T. J. (1979). *Smallholder marketing in Kenya*. Nairobi: Central Bureau of Statistics.

Clapp, J., & Fuchs, D. (2009). Agrifood corporations, global governance, and sustainability: A framework for analysis. In J. Clapp & D. Fuchs (Eds.), *Corporate power in global agrifood governance* (pp. 2–26). Cambridge: Massachusetts Institute of Technology.

Cowen, M. P., & Shenton, R. W. (1996). *Doctrines of development*. London: Routledge.

Creamy Inn. (2011). *Dial a delivery: Great choice in motion, step 2*. Retrieved from http://dialadeliverykenya.co.ke/creamyinn

Daily Nation. (2014a). Roof-high interest rates put ceiling to real estate growth. Retrieved from http://www.nation.co.ke/business/Roof-high-interest-rates-put-ceiling-to-real-estate-growth/-/996/2267428/-/qf3sexz/-/index.html

Daily Nation. (2014b). It's worth it: Beauty firms chase Africa cosmetics boom. Retrieved from http://www.nation.co.ke/lifestyle/beauty/beauty/Africa-cosmetics-boom/-/2115038/2265666/-/x2udbaz/-/index.html

David, H. (2014). Pepsi coke replaces Kenya chief in battle with coke. *Daily Nation*. Retrieved from http://www.nation.co.ke/business/PepsiCo-replaces-Kenya-chief-in-battle-with-Coke/-/996/2152744/-/13cjvlnz/-/index.html

Daviron, B. (2008). The historical integration of Africa in the international food trade: A food regime perspective. In N. Fold & M. Nylandsted Larsen (Eds.), *Globalization and restructuring of African commodity flows* (pp. 44–78). Uppsala: Nordiska Afrikainstitutet.

De Vogli, R., Kouvonen, A., & Gimeno, D. (2011). 'Globesization': Ecological evidence on the relationship between fast food outlets and obesity among 26 advanced economies. *Critical Public Health, 21*, 395–402.

Delgado, C. L. (2003). Rising consumption of meat and milk in developing countries has created a new food revolution. *The Journal of Nutrition, 133*, 3907S–3910S.

Dinham, B., & Hines, C. (1984). *Agribusiness in Africa*. Trenton, NJ: Africa World Press.

Drewnowski, A., & Popkin, B. M. (1997). The Nutrition transition: New trends in the global diet. *Nutrition Reviews, 55*, 31–43.

Export Processing Zones Authority Kenya. (2005). *Vegetable oil industry in Kenya*. Retrieved from http://www.epzakenya.com/UserFiles/File/kenyaVegetableOil.pdf

FAO. (2014). *Interactive hunger map*. Retrieved from http://www.fao.org/hunger/en/

FAOSTAT. (2014a). *Food balance, food supply*. Retrieved from http://faostat.fao.org/site/345/default.aspx

FAOSTAT. (2014b). *Production, crops*. Retrieved from http://faostat.fao.org/site/567/default.aspx#ancor

FAOSTAT. (2014c). *Trade, detailed trade flows*. Retrieved from http://faostat.fao.org/DesktopModules/Faostat/WATFDetailed2/watf.aspx?PageID=536

Farmer, E., & Mbwika, J. (2012). *End market analysis of Kenyan livestock and meat* (microReport No. 184). Retrieved from https://www.microlinks.org/library/end-market-analysis-kenyan-livestock-and-meat-desk-study

Friedmann, H. (1992). Distance and durability: Shaky foundations of the world food economy. *Third World Quarterly, 13*, 371–383.

Friedmann, H. (1999). Remaking 'Traditions': How we eat, what we eat and the changing political economy of food. In D. Barndt (Ed.), *Women working the NAFTA food chain: Women, food & globalization* (pp. 36–60). Toronto: Sumach Press.

Friedmann, H., & McMichael, P. (1989). Agriculture and the state system: The rise and decline of national agricultures, 1870 to the present. *Sociologia Ruralis, 29*, 93–117.

Friedmann, H. (2005). From colonialism to green capitalism: Social movements and emergence of food regimes. In F. H. Buttel & P. McMichael (Eds.), *New directions in the sociology of global development* (pp. 227–264). Bingley: Emerald Group.

Friel, S., Hattersley, L., Snowdon, W., Thow, A.-M., Lobstein, T., Sanders, D., … Walker, C. (2013). Monitoring the impacts of trade agreements on food environments. *Obesity Reviews, 14*, 120–134.

Galito's. (2011). *Some words about us.* Retrieved from http://www.galitoschicken.com/about_us.php

Gereffi, G., & Christian, M. (2010). Trade, transnational corporations and food consumption: A global value chain approach. In C. Hawkes, C. Blouin, S. Henson, N. Drager, & L. Dubée (Eds.), *Trade, food, diet and health* (pp. 91–109). Oxford: Wiley-Blackwell.

Gibendi, R. (2013). Egyptian poultry firm plans Kenyan entry. *Daily Nation.* Retrieved from http://www.nation.co.ke/lifestyle/smartcompany/Egyptian-poultry-firm-plans-Kenyan-entry/-/1226/1959952/-/bh8fv8/-/index.html

Gibendi, R. (2014a). Sugar: Comesa gives Kenya time. *Daily Nation.* Retrieved from http://www.nation.co.ke/news/Sugar-Comesa-gives-Kenya-time/-/1056/2223548/-/k09cdaz/-/index.html

Gibendi, R. (2014b). Team named to reform parastatals. *Daily Nation.* Retrieved from http://www.nation.co.ke/business/Team-named-to-reform-parastatals/-/996/2246044/-/7j6pon/-/index.html

Gikunju, W. (2013). The Pepsi challenge – Drinks giant returns to Kenya after 40 years. *The South African.* Retrieved from http://www.thesouthafrican.com/featured/the-pepsi-challenge-drinks-giant-returns-to-kenya-after-40-years.htm

Government of Kenya. (1965). *African socialism and its application to planning in Kenya.* Nairobi: Government of Kenya.

Government of Kenya. (2009). *Price control act.* Nairobi: Government of Kenya.

Hawkes, C. (2005). The role of foreign direct investment in the nutrition transition. *Public Health Nutrition, 8*, 357–365.

Hawkes, C. (2006). Uneven dietary development: Linking the policies and processes of globalization with the nutrition transition, obesity and diet-related chronic diseases. *Globalization and Health, 2*, 4. doi:10.1186/1744-8603

Hawkes, C. (2010). The influence of trade liberalisation and global dietary change: The case of vegetable oils, meat and highly processed foods. In C. Hawkes, C. Blouin, S. Henson, N. Drager, & L. Dubée (Eds.), *Trade, food, diet and health* (pp. 35–59). Oxford: Wiley-Blackwell.

Hebinck, P. G. M. (1990). *The Agrarian structure in Kenya: State, farmers and commodity relations.* Verlag: Breitenbach.

Jabara, C. L. (1985). Agricultural pricing policy in Kenya. *World Development, 13*, 611–626.

Kabukuru, W. (2009, May). When Kenya sneezes. *New African,* p. 64.

Kenchic. (2012). *About us.* Retrieved from http://www.kenchic.com/about-us

Kenya Meat Commission. (2014). *Market.* Retrieved from http://www.kenyameat.co.ke/index.php?option=com_content&view=category&layout=blog&id=37&Itemid=69

Leys, C. (1975). *Underdevelopment in Kenya.* London: Heinemann.

Maina, W. (2012). Kenafric chews into the market with a sweet Sh1 billion confectionary plant. *Business Daily.* Retrieved from http://www.businessdailyafrica.com/Corporate-News/Kenafric-launches-Sh1bn-confectionary-plant/-/539550/1531456/-/1270o9ez/-/index.html

Maina, W. (2014). Java, Subway eye middle class cash with new outlets. *Daily Nation.* Retrieved from http://www.nation.co.ke/business/corporates/Java-Subway-/-/1954162/2266646/-/ihjqjdz/-/index.html

Matejowsky, T. (2009). Fast food and nutritional perceptions in the age of "Globesity": Perspectives from the provincial Philippines. *Food and Foodways, 17*, 29–49.

Maxon, R. M. (1992). Small-scale and large-scale agriculture since independence. In W. R. Ochieng' & R. M. Maxon (Eds.), *An economic history of Kenya* (pp. 273–296). Nairobi: East African Educational Publishers Ltd.

McMichael, P. (2005). Global development and the corporate food regime. In F. H. Buttel & P. McMichael (Eds.), *New directions in the sociology of global development* (pp. 265–299). Bingley: Emerald.

McMichael, P. (2009). A food regime genealogy. *Journal of Peasant Studies, 36*, 139–169.

Mendez, M. A., Montiero, C. A., & Popkin, B. M. (2005). Overweight exceeds underweight among women in most developing countries. *The American Journal of Clinical Nutrition, 81*, 714–721.

Ministry of Finance and Economic Planning. (1971). *Statistical abstract of Kenya.* Nairobi: Central of Bureau of Statistics.

Muraya, J. W. (2014). Experts raise alarm over rising number of fat children in towns. *Daily Nation.* Retrieved from http://www.nation.co.ke/news/Experts-raise-alarm-over-rising-number-of-fat-children-in-towns/-/1056/2272100/-/l63ajk/-/index.html

Muyanga, M., Jayne, T. S., Argwings-Kodhek, G., & Ariga, J. (2005). *Staple food consumption patterns in urban Kenya: Trends and policy implications* (Working Paper 19). Nairobi: Tegemeo Institute of Agricultural Policy and Development, Egerton University. Retrieved from http://www.tegemeo.org/images/downloads/Working%20papers/tegemeo_workingpaper_19.pdf

Ndemwa, P. (2013). Lifestyle diseases like obesity can be controlled by simple exercise and diet. *Daily Nation.* Retrieved from http://www.nation.co.ke/oped/Opinion//440808/1905046/-/j2seh1z/-/index.html

Nestle, M. (2002/2013). *Food politics: How the food industry influences nutrition and health.* Berkeley: University of California Press.

Neven, D., & Reardon, T. (2004). The rise of Kenyan supermarkets and the evolution of their horticulture product procurement systems. *Development Policy Review, 22*, 669–699.

Neven, D., Reardon, T., Chege, J., & Wang, H. (2006). Supermarkets and consumers in Africa: The case of Nairobi, Kenya. *Journal of International Food and Agribusiness Marketing, 18*, 103–123.

Neven, D., Odera, M. M., Reardon, T., & Wang, H. (2009). Kenyan supermarkets, emerging middle-class horticultural farmers, and employment impacts on the rural poor. *World Development, 37*, 1802–1811.

Ngwiri, M. (2014). Let's cut out the sugar and fats from our diet to fight obesity. *Daily Nation.* Retrieved from http://www.nation.co.ke/oped/Opinion/cut-out-the-sugar-and-fat-from-our-diets/-/440808/2141572/-/156w5qaz/-/index.html

Nyangito, H. O., Nzuma, J., Ommeh, H., & Mbithi, M. (2006). Kenya. In H. Thomas (Ed.), *Trade reforms and food security* (pp. 365–398). Rome: Food and Agriculture Organization of the United Nations.

Ochieng', W. R. (1992). The post-colonial state and Kenya's economic inheritance. In W. R. Ochieng' & R. M. Maxon (Eds.), *An economic history of Kenya* (pp. 259–272). Nairobi: East African Educational Publishers Ltd.

Odame, H., Musyoka, P., & Kere, J. (2009). Kenya: Maize, tomato, and dairy. In K. Larsen, R. Kim, & F. Theus (Eds.), *Agribusiness and innovation systems in Africa* (pp. 89–134). Washington, DC: World Bank.

Okeyo, V. (2012). Swiss firm set to raise the bar in chocolate market. *Business Daily.* Retrieved from http://www.businessdailyafrica.com/Swiss-firm-set-to-raise-the-bar-in-chocolate-market/-/1248928/1528204/-/b6ne2z/-/index.html

Otero, G., Pechlaner, G., & Gürcan, E. (2013). The political economy of "food security" and trade: Uneven and combined dependency. *Rural Sociology, 78*, 263–289.

Otieno, R. (2013). *Coca-Cola marks Kenya @50 with Sh100 m sponsorship deal.* Retrieved from https://www.standardmedia.co.ke/business/article/2000098796/coca-cola-marks-kenya-50-with-sh100 m-sponsorship-deal

Patel, R. (2007). *Stuffed and starved: The hidden battle for the world's food system*. London: Portobello Books.

Pechlaner, G., & Otero, G. (2010). The Neoliberal food regime: Neoregulation and the new division of labor in North America. *Rural Sociology, 75*, 179–208.

Pizza Inn. (2013). *Pizza Inn menu*. Retrieved from http://www.thejunction.co.ke/our-stores/store-directory/by-alphabetical/item/219-pizza-inn

Popkin, B. M. (1993). Nutritional patterns and transitions. *Population and Development Review, 19*, 138–157.

Popkin, B. M. (1994). The nutrition transition in low-income countries: An emerging crisis. *Nutrition Reviews, 52*, 285–298.

Popkin, B. M. (2006). Technology, transport, globalization and the nutrition transition food policy. *Food Policy, 31*, 554–569.

Raschke, V., & Cheema, B. (2008). Colonisation, the new world order, and the eradication of traditional food habits in East Africa: Historical perspective on the nutrition transition. *Public Health Nutrition, 11*, 662–674.

Ravallion, M. (2009). The developing world's bulging (but vulnerable) middle class. *World Development, 38*, 445–454.

Ritzer, G. (2006). *McDonaldization: The reader* (2nd ed.). Thousand Oaks: Pine Forge Press.

Stanford, D. (2010). *Africa: Coke's last frontier*. Retrieved from http://www.businessweek.com/magazine/content/10_45/b4202054144294.htm

Steers. (2014a). *Family meal packs*. Retrieved from http://steers.co.ke/

Steers. (2014b). *Menu – Burgers*. Retrieved from http://steers.co.ke/menu/burgers/

Steyn, N. P., Nel, J. H., Parker, W., Ayah, R., & Mbithe, D. (2012). Urbanisation and the nutrition transition: A comparison of diet and weight status of South African and Kenyan women. *Scandinavian Journal of Public Health, 40*, 229–238.

Stuckler, D., & Nestle, M. (2012). Big food, food systems, and global health. *PLOS Medicine, 9*, e1001242. doi:10.1371/journal.pmed.1001242

Swainson, N. (1980). *The development of corporate capitalism in Kenya, 1918–1977*. Berkeley: University of California Press.

Swamy, G. (1994). *Kenya: Structural adjustment in the 1980s*. Washington, DC: Chief Economist's Office, Africa Regional Office. Retrieved from http://wwwds.worldbank.org/servlet/WDSContentServer/WDSP/IB/1994/01/01/000009265_3961005201828/Rendered/PDF/multi0page.pdf

Swynnerton, R. J. M. (1954). *Plan to intensify the development of African agriculture in Kenya*. Nairobi: Government of Kenya.

Thow, A.-M., & Hawkes, C. (2009). The implications of trade liberalization for diet and health: A case study from central America. *Globalization and Health, 5*, 5. doi:10.1186/1744-8603-5-5

Unilever. (2014). *Brands in action: Blue band, Rama*. Retrieved from http://www.unilever.com/brands-in-action/detail/Blue-Band–Rama/292005/

Vorster, H. H., Kruger, A., & Margetts, B. M. (2011). The nutrition transition in Africa: Can it be steered into a more positive direction? *Nutrients, 3*, 429–441.

Wanja, J. (2010). Kenya`s new silent killer. *Daily Nation*. Retrieved from http://www.nation.co.ke/lifestyle/Kenyas-silent-killer-/-/1190/1013946/-/24xal4/-/index.html

Weis, T. (2007). *The global food economy: The battle for the future of farming*. New York, NY: Zed Books.

Winter-Nelson, A. (1995). A history of agricultural policy in Kenya. In S. R. Pearson & E. A. Monke (Eds.), *Agricultural policy in Kenya* (pp. 31–48). Ithaca: Cornell University Press.

World Health Organization. (2011). *Global database on body mass index*. Retrieved from http://apps.who.int/bmi/index.jsp

WTO. (2013). *Regional trade agreements: Scope of RTAs*. Retrieved from http://www.wto.org/english/tratop_e/region_e/scope_rta_e.htm

Density of outdoor food and beverage advertising around schools in Ulaanbaatar (Mongolia) and Manila (The Philippines) and implications for policy

Bridget Kelly[a], Lesley King[b], Batjargal Jamiyan[c], Nyamragchaa Chimedtseren[c], Bolorchimeg Bold[d], Victoria M. Medina[e], Sarah J. De los Reyes[f], Nichel V. Marquez[g], Anna Christine P. Rome[h,i], Ariane Margareth O. Cabanes[j], John Juliard Go[k], Tsogzolmaa Bayandorj[l], Marie Clem B. Carlos[m] and Cherian Varghese[m]

[a]Early Start Research Institute, School of Health and Society, University of Wollongong, Wollongong, Australia; [b]Prevention Research Collaboration, Sydney School of Public Health, University of Sydney, Sydney, Australia; [c]Nutrition Research Department, National Center for Public Health, Ulaanbaatar, Mongolia; [d]Ministry of Health, Ulaanbaatar, Mongolia; [e]Institute of Community and Family Health Inc., Quezon City, The Philippines; [f]Dr. Fe Del Mundo Medical Center, Quezon City, The Philippines; [g]Activeone Health Inc, Manila, The Philippines; [h]Independent Research Assistant, Manila, The Philippines; [i]College of Home Economics, University of the Philippines, Manila, The Philippines; [j]Independent Advertising Consultant, Manila, The Philippines; [k]World Health Organization Representative Office in the Philippines, Manila, The Philippines; [l]World Health Organization Representative Office in Mongolia, Ulaanbaatar, Mongolia; [m]Noncommunicable Diseases and Health Promotion, World Health Organization, Regional Office for the Western Pacific, Manila, The Philippines

Children's exposure to unhealthy food marketing is recognised by leading international health organisations as a probable causal factor for obesity. Outdoor advertising near schools embeds commercial food messages into children's everyday lives and acts as a cue for food purchases. This project aimed to describe food advertising in the area around schools in two demographically and culturally disparate cities in the Asia Pacific Region. Data on outdoor food advertising were collected from the area within 500 m of 30 primary schools in each of two cities: Ulaanbaatar, Mongolia and Manila, The Philippines. For each food advertisement, information was collected on: distance from the school (within 250 or 500 m); size, setting, type and position of the advertisement; and the food/drink product type promoted (core/healthy, non-core/unhealthy and miscellaneous). Density of advertisements was calculated per 100 m². The density of food advertising was twice as high in the area closest to schools compared to the area further from schools (.9 vs. .5 in Ulaanbaatar and 6.5 vs. 3.3 advertisements per 100 m² in Manila). Almost all food advertisements were for non-core/unhealthy foods/drinks (92% in Ulaanbaatar and 85% in Manila), and soft drinks were most frequently promoted. Children in Ulaanbaatar and Manila are exposed to large numbers of advertisements for unhealthy foods/drinks on their way to and from school, and these are particularly clustered within the immediate vicinity of schools. Clear directions for policy development are outlined to reduce children's exposure to this marketing, including restricting the placement and content of outdoor advertising.

Introduction

Unhealthy diet is a significant and modifiable risk factor for non-communicable diseases (NCDs), and improving population nutrition is a key NCD prevention strategy (World Health Organization, 2004). Improving population nutrition involves comprehensive strategies to encourage and support reduced consumption of energy-dense, nutrient-poor (EDNP) foods and non-alcoholic beverages, including environmental changes to reduce availability and cues for consumption of these foods. As presented in the *Global Strategy on Diet, Physical Activity and Health,* one component of a comprehensive approach comprises reducing the marketing of EDNP foods and non-alcoholic beverages (World Health Organization, 2004). In 2010, the World Health Assembly endorsed a set of recommendations on the marketing of foods and non-alcoholic beverages to children (World Health Organization, 2010). These recommendations aim to guide Member States in developing new and/or strengthening existing policies on food and non-alcoholic beverage marketing to children.

Internationally, there is an accumulating body of research on the nature and extent of food marketing to children, indicating the predominance of marketing for EDNP foods and beverages. While most studies, to date, have focused on television, food marketing is widespread across other media. Outdoor advertising in particular works by integrating branded messages into daily activities and the cultural landscape, and also serves as an immediate cue for purchase when this is viewed in connection with food stores (Kelly et al., in press). There have been four published studies specifically on outdoor food advertising: one study from Sydney, Australia (Kelly, Cretikos, Rogers, & King, 2008), one conducted in four cities in the USA (Hillier et al., 2009), one in Northern England (Adams, Ganiti, & White, 2011), and a fourth in Wellington, New Zealand (Walton, Pearce, & Day, 2009). These studies have consistently found that the majority of outdoor food advertisements are for unhealthy foods/drinks, and that the density of advertisements varies by neighbourhood characteristics. Two of these studies (from Australia and New Zealand) have examined the area around schools and found unhealthy food marketing to be prevalent in the vicinity of schools (Kelly et al., 2008; Walton et al., 2009). While information on the prevalence of food and beverage marketing in low- and middle-income countries is limited, with only a few studies available that measured advertising on television (Consumers International, 2008; Kelly et al., 2010), it has been suggested that children in developing countries may be more vulnerable to food promotion because they have been traditionally less familiar with, and potentially less critical of, advertising (Hastings, McDermott, Angus, Stead, & Thomson, 2006).

To contribute to the process for implementing the *Global Strategy on Diet, Physical Activity and Health* (World Health Organization, 2004) and the WHO set of recommendations on food marketing to children (World Health Organization, 2010), health professionals in a number of countries raised concerns about the prevalence of unhealthy food advertising around schools at a regional consultation meeting convened by WHO (World Health Organization Western Pacific Region, 2012). As part of a suite of actions with potential to promote children's nutrition, the meeting identified the need for local information on the extent and nature of food marketing, in order to guide locally relevant and feasible policy actions. In particular, government delegates from Mongolia and The Philippines initiated an assessment of outdoor advertising around schools, in collaboration with the regional office of the WHO. In both of these countries, there was no information available on the extent of children's exposure to food and beverage marketing generally, including outdoor advertising, which is required to guide any policy in this area.

The aims of each country-based project were to identify, describe and quantify the volume of food and beverage advertisements around schools; with projects conducted in the capital city of each of these two demographically and culturally disparate cities in Asia. Information on the volume of unhealthy food and beverage advertisements in the area near primary schools provides an indication of the extent of children's exposure to this form of marketing and the need for policy interventions. Specific information on the types of products promoted and the nature of these promotions, including their format and placement, are necessary to inform any regulations or guidelines in this area.

Methods

Sampled sites

Data were collected in two cities: Ulaanbaatar (Mongolia) and Manila (The Philippines). In each city, 30 primary schools (public and private) were randomly selected from lists of all schools within sampled areas ($N = 200$ in Ulaanbaatar and 156 in Manila). Where the study area of two schools overlapped, a replacement school was identified. In Ulaanbaatar, schools were selected from six districts, covering all of the main city areas. Five schools from each district were included: three schools from 'apartment areas' and two schools from 'ger areas'. Apartment areas located in the central area of the city, have a higher population density and are wealthier. Ger areas comprise those locations with traditional housing and lower density, and relatively lower socio-economic status (Kamata, Reichert, Tsevegmid, Yoonhee, & Sedgewick, 2010). In Manila, schools were selected from four cities within the Greater Manila area: Las Pinas, Makati, Manila and Marikina, and the municipality of Taytay in Rizal Province. The distribution of 'poverty incidence' across these areas ranges from 1.4% in Makati to 3.2% in Taytay (Philippine Statistics Authority, 2009). Poverty incidence refers to the proportion of households with per capita income/expenditure less than the minimum income/expenditure required for a family/individual to meet the basic food and non-food requirements. Four public and two private schools were randomly selected within each city/municipality.

Data collection and coding

An 'advertisement' was defined as signs with branded information, pictures or logos. This included billboards, posters, free standing signs, neon signs, stickers, electronic boards, banners, bus shelter signs and signs on outdoor furniture, bridge/awning signs and painted buildings. Signage, defined as symbols or words that are used mainly for store identification, were excluded. However, store signage that also had a product logo and served not just as a store identifier but also as promotional material for a product, was considered as an advertisement. All branded references to food and drink products that fitted the above specifications were considered to be food advertisements.

For each school, a map was generated using Google Maps, with concentric circles marked to indicate the distance within 250 and 500 m from the centre of the school property. All streets within these radii of selected schools were surveyed. In each country, surveys were conducted by three teams, each comprising two locally recruited members.

A standard template for recording the outdoor food and drink advertisements was used. The information collected comprised: distance of food/drink advertisement from school (within 250 or 500 m); size of advertisement (small ($\geq$21 cm $\times$ 30 cm but <1.3 m $\times$ 1.9 m); medium ($\geq$1.3 m $\times$ 1.9 m but <2.0 m $\times$ 2.5 m); and large ($\geq$2 m $\times$ 2.5 m)); setting of advertisement (shop, street, etc.); type and position of advertisement (neon sign, billboard, etc.); whether the subject of the advertisement was single or multiple foods; and food/drink brand name and product type.

Advertised foods and drinks were classified as core/healthy, non-core/unhealthy and miscellaneous based on a classification system used in previous research on outdoor advertising (Kelly et al., 2008) and international research on television food advertising (Kelly et al., 2010). This classification system was refined to include a wider range of traditional Asian foods available in Mongolia and The Philippines (Table 2).

In each country, a pilot survey was conducted as part of the training for field teams, and to check coding reliability. Responses by the principal investigator were compared to all other research assistants individually. Inter-rater reliability ranged from 40 to 80% (Mongolia) and from 54 to 86% (The Philippines). Further training was provided to field teams in Mongolia and data collectors were paired to maximise the reliability of data collection. In The Philippines, training was followed by a review and discussion of the pilot survey coding. Data collection ran from 21 to 30 May 2012 (Mongolia) and from 13 to 25 August 2012 (The Philippines).

Data analysis

Data were entered into SPSS for Windows version 17.0 (SPSS Inc., Chicago, IL) and Stata version 10 (StataCorp LP., College Station, TX) by research groups in each country and checked for data entry errors by the lead researchers at each site. For each country, two data-sets were generated: one related to the advertisements observed, and one for the food products depicted in the advertisements (as some advertisements promoted more than one product type). Density of advertisements were calculated per 100 m², to enable standardised comparisons of advertising rates in the area closest to, and further away, from schools. For each site, descriptive analyses were conducted to determine the frequency of food/drink advertisements by school areas, product type, location and type and size of advertisements.

Results

Mongolia

A total of 1459 food and beverage advertisements were identified in the area around sampled schools. Most outdoor advertisements featured a single food product, although 11% of advertisements promoted two or more branded food products, and single advertisements were found to promote up to 24 products.

The mean number of food advertisements within 250 m of each school was 18, compared to 31 advertisements in the area further from schools. However, while there were more food advertisements in the area between 250 and 500 m from schools, the density of food advertisements was .9 ads/100 m² in the area closest to schools (up to 250 m) compared to .5 ads/100 m² in the area 250–500 m from schools (Table 1). The overall density of food and beverage advertisements was more than twice as high in

Table 1. Mean number of food advertisements per school and per 100 m^2, by distance from school and high/low population density areas.

Demographic area	Mean (ads/100 m^2) food ads <250 m from schools	Mean (ads/100 m^2) food ads 250–500 m from school	Mean total food ads (ads/100 m^2)
Mongolia	18 (.9)	31 (.5)	49 (.6)
Ger (low density)	11 (.6)	13 (.2)	25 (.3)
Apartment (high density)	22 (1.1)	42 (.7)	65 (.8)
Philippines	128 (6.5)	195 (3.3)	323 (4.1)
Makati (high density)	202 (10.3)	291 (4.9)	494 (6.3)
Manila (high density)	130 (6.6)	293 (5.0)	424 (5.4)
Marikina (high density)	112 (5.7)	141 (2.4)	253 (3.2)
Las Piñas (low density)	59 (3.0)	90 (1.5)	149 (1.9)
Taytay (low density)	136 (6.9)	158 (2.7)	294 (3.8)

Apartment areas, which have a greater population density and less social disadvantage, compared to Ger areas.

Most food advertisements were located in shopping areas (59%), or attached to restaurants or cafes (17%). In terms of display type, most advertisements were on awnings (46%), such as above shop entrances or on billboards (25%). Half of all advertisements were medium in size, while 34% were large and 16% were small.

Types of advertised foods and beverages

Most advertised products were non-core food/drinks (92%) (Table 2), with an average of 66 non-core products advertised around each school (Table 3). This pattern of predominantly non-core food advertising was found across all school districts, ger and apartment areas, across settings and positions, and regardless of advertisement size. The food and beverage types most commonly advertised were sugar-sweetened drinks (52%) followed by fruit juice/drinks (10%). Coca Cola (35%) and Pepsi (10%) were the food/drink brands most commonly advertised.

The Philippines

A total of 9687 food advertisements were identified around sampled schools. Again, the density of advertising was highest in the area closest to schools, with 6.5 advertisements per 100 m^2 compared to 3.3 per 100 m^2 in the area between 250 and 500 m from schools (Table 1). The mean number of food advertisements within 250 m of each school was 128, compared to 195 advertisements in the area further from schools.

Table 2. Frequency of promoted foods and beverages.

	Mongolia, n (%)	Philippines, n (%)
Core foods	148 (7)	463 (5)
Plain bread and cereal products	62 (3)	142 (1)
Bottled water	22 (1)	105 (1)
Meat and meat alternatives	13 (1)	105 (1)
Healthy oils and low fat savoury sauces	14 (1)	0 (0)
Low fat dairy and alternatives, and probiotic drinks	11 (1)	76 (1)
Fruits	12 (1)	12 (0)
Low fat/salt meals	12 (1)	12 (0)
Baby foods	2 (0)	3 (0)
Vegetables	0 (0)	8 (0)
Non-core foods	1975 (92)	8469 (85)
Sugar sweetened drinks	1115 (52)	5612 (56)
Fruit juice/drinks	207 (10)	596 (6)
Fast food	110 (5)	449 (5)
Processed meat/alternatives	106 (5)	218 (2)
Chocolate and candy	101 (5)	0 (0)
Sweet breads, glutinous rice, pies and pastries	78 (4)	0 (0)
Ice cream	29 (1)	640 (6)
Other non-core drinks	0 (0)	139 (1)
Other non-core foods	144 (6)	107 (1)
Alcohol	85 (4)	708 (7)
Miscellaneous	14 (1)	1004 (10)
Restaurant (not fast food) and coffee shops	0 (0)	252 (2)
Tea and coffee	2 (0)	111 (1)
Convenience store	0 (0)	80 (1)
Food supplement	0 (0)	73 (1)
Condiments, seasonings and recipe additions	11 (1)	37 (0)
Baby and toddler milk formulae	1 (0)	0 (0)
Total	2137 (100)	9936 (100)

Note: Some advertisements depicted more than one food or beverage product.

Table 3. Mean number of food products promoted per school and per $100 \, m^2$, by distance from school and food category.

Site	Mean (per $100 \, m^2$) food products promoted <250 m from schools	Mean (per $100 \, m^2$) food products promoted 250–500 m from schools	Mean total products promoted (per $100 \, m^2$)
Mongolia			
Core	2 (.1)	3 (.1)	5 (.1)
Non-core	24 (1.2)	42 (.7)	66 (.8)
Miscellaneous	<1 (.0)	<1 (.0)	1 (.0)
Philippines			
Core	6 (.3)	10 (.2)	15 (.2)
Non-core	115 (5.8)	168 (2.8)	282 (3.7)
Miscellaneous	12 (.6)	22 (.4)	33 (.4)

Note: Some advertisements depicted more than one food or beverage product.

Most advertisements were small in size (86%), located in shopping areas (defined as a cluster of at least five stores) (86%), and promoted a single product (99%). Advertisements were mostly in the form of banners (32%), posters (29%), store signage with a brand logo (26%) and in-store merchandising (e.g. branded refrigerators, bins, chairs and umbrellas) (9%).

Types of advertised foods and beverages

The majority of advertised foods/drinks were non-core (85%), with an average of 282 non-core food/drink products promoted in the area around each school. Non-core product promotions were more densely displayed in the area closest to schools (Table 3). More than half of non-core food/drink promotions were for sugar-sweetened drinks (Table 2). Of these advertised drinks, soft drinks comprised 83%, energy drinks 14% and sweetened tea 3%. The most frequently promoted brand was Coca Cola (32% of all promotions), followed by a local soft drink manufacturer, RC Cola (8%). The density of non-core food/drink promotions was higher around private schools (4.4 promotions per 100 m^2 vs. 3.2 for public schools).

Discussion

The vast majority of foods and beverage advertisements around schools in Ulaanbaatar, Mongolia and Manila, The Philippines were for non-core products (92 and 85%, respectively). This is similar to the proportion of these non-core products promoted on food advertisements in Sydney (80%) (Kelly et al., 2008), and in the UK, where only 11% of food advertising space (frequency × size of all food advertisements) was for core food products (Adams et al., 2011).

The density of food advertising in the immediate area of schools, within 250 m, was almost double that in the area further away from schools (.9 vs. .5 in Ulaanbaatar and 6.5 vs. 3.3 advertisements per 100 m^2 in Manila). Similar patterns were observed in an earlier study in Sydney, Australia using a similar methodology (1.2 vs. .6) (Kelly et al., 2008). While in each location, there were larger numbers of food and beverage advertisements in areas within 250 and 500 m from schools, this comprised an area three times larger than the area within 250 m of schools. The density of food advertising around schools is of concern in both Manila and Ulaanbaatar. However, food advertising density was particularly high in Manila, with an average of 323 food advertisements within 500 m of each school. This compares to an average of 49 food advertisements per school in Ulaanbaatar and 57 per school in Sydney (Kelly et al., 2008). This type of monitoring data on food marketing is necessary for determining the extent and nature of current marketing to children, and for identifying priority areas for policy action (World Health Organization, 2012). This data will be useful in contributing to the International Network for Food and Obesity/non-communicable diseases Research, Monitoring and Action Support (INFORMAS) initiative, which aims to monitor and benchmark countries in aspects of food environments, including food marketing, and ultimately develop a global database to assess changes to these environments over time and across regions (Swinburn et al., 2013).

This study has demonstrated that unhealthy food and beverage advertisements are highly prevalent around schools and are particularly dense in the immediate vicinity of schools (within 250 m). This means that children are repeatedly and frequently exposed to these advertisements each school day on their way to and from school. Outdoor advertising provides cues for the purchase and consumption of products, and makes the brands and products highly familiar and desirable to children. For example, one study from the USA found that sixth-grade children who were exposed to advertisements for alcoholic beverages within 1500 ft of their schools were more likely to have positive attitudes and behaviours about drinking when they reached the eighth grade (Pasch, Komro, Perry, Hearst, & Farbakhsh, 2007). The prevalence of advertising for alcoholic beverages near schools (7% of all promoted products in Manila and 4% in Ulaanbaatar) is of particular concern. Similarly, given efforts to include nutrition education in school curricula, and to disseminate healthy eating guidelines to community members in both of the study countries (World Health Organization Western Pacific Region, 2012), the frequent exposure to advertisements for unhealthy foods can be seen as contradicting and undermining educational initiatives.

In both Manila and Ulaanbaatar, soft drinks were the most heavily promoted products in the area around schools, with the majority of advertised products were from one large multi-national company. Sugar-sweetened soft drinks have been identified by the WHO as a probable causal factor in weight gain and obesity (World Health Organization, 2003).

A large proportion of food advertisements in this study was found around shops and commercial areas near schools, where advertising is used to promote the products that are available in-store. Outdoor food advertising appears to be closely associated with the population density of areas and the presence of shops. These findings are congruous with other studies which had found clustering of advertising around high traffic areas. Hillier et al. (2009) found that land use variables, such as major streets, shops and bus stops explained some of the clustering around child-institutions, and that variations between cities were partially explained by land use and outdoor advertising regulations. In Ulaanbaatar, these high population density areas were also those areas of lower social disadvantage. That is, were apartment building existed rather than traditional Ger housing. These observations are aligned with disease patterns in developing countries, where increasing wealth is associated with 'Westernised' and higher fat diets (Stuckler, McKee, Ebrahim, & Basu, 2012).

Land use regulations, including zoning, offer a key tool for limiting children's exposure to unhealthy food advertising. While mixed land use may be desirable for promoting active travel, the co-location of shops and schools appears to be associated with high exposure to unhealthy food and beverage advertising. Advertising regulations may apply to off-premise (not located on shops) and on-premise signage and advertising. In the USA, since 2008 Los Angeles has prohibited any new off-premise billboards, while Austin has banned any new billboards since 1983 (Hillier et al., 2009). While the majority of food advertisements in Manila and Ulaanbaatar comprised on-premise advertising, in the form of branded store signage, posters and branded merchandise, there is still clearly scope for these jurisdictions to adopt similar regulations to control outdoor off-license advertising as a starting point.

Current marketing regulations in both Mongolia and The Philippines are inadequate in limiting children's exposure to outdoor advertising for unhealthy foods and beverages. In The Philippines, industry self-regulatory pledges only make provisions to preclude the promotion of products or services that are not suitable for children or which might cause them physical, mental, psychological or moral harm from being broadcast in or adjacent to children's television programmes (Outdoor Advertising Association of the Philippines, 2006). No specific regulations relating to the content and volume of outdoor food advertising near and around schools are available. By comparison, no specific government or industry regulations on food marketing exist in Mongolia. While international industry pledges exist, such as from the International Council of Beverages Associations Council's Marketing to Children Guidelines (ICBA Pledge) and the International Food and Beverage Alliance Global Policy on Marketing and Advertising to Children (IFBA Pledge), these do not apply to outdoor advertising (Yale Rudd Center for Food Policy and Obesity, 2013).

Policies in Mongolia and The Philippines could focus on introducing regulations related to higher population density areas, including apartment areas in Ulaanbaatar and urbanised cities in Manila. The proposal to limit unhealthy food advertising around schools is consistent with the 'green food zone' operating in South Korea, which involves limiting the availability and advertising of unhealthy foods within 200 m from schools (Korean Ministry of Food and Drug Safety, 2010). Such regulations to limit outdoor advertising of unhealthy foods could be integrated into development plans and urban planning initiatives. The Health Promoting School concept and the WHO School Policy Framework (World Health Organization, 2008) also suggest taking measures to create a supportive environment in the area around schools, by limiting the availability of unhealthy foods and drinks in these vicinities. Outdoor food marketing also has relevance to the WHO concept of 'Healthy Cities', which seeks to encourage inter-sectoral health promotion efforts to create social, physical and economic environments conducive to health on an urban scale, and encompasses the extent to which physical infrastructure supports health (Flynn, 1996). Thus, outdoor advertising of unhealthy foods is inconsistent with the basic premise and aim of Healthy Cities. It is recommended that any policies to reduce unhealthy food advertising encompass a comprehensive range of food products high in sugar, fat and salt. However, the predominance of advertising for sugar-sweetened drinks suggests that reducing children's exposure to these advertisements is a priority.

Policies that limit the promotion of unhealthy food and beverages, including outdoor advertising, should be supported by broader synergistic regulations to decrease the accessibility of unhealthy choices, such as sugary drinks. For example, introducing taxes on sugary drinks may reduce demand for these products (Cabrera Escobar, Veerman, Tollman, Bertram, & Hofman, 2013). Zoning regulations could also limit the placement of food outlets selling unhealthy foods, such as fast food restaurants, from the area around schools, given that these outlets have been associated with higher consumption of sugary drinks and greater odds of obesity (Davis & Carpenter, 2009). School policies should support the availability and promotion of healthy food and beverage choices within school grounds, with Japan and Hong Kong providing good examples of how these school policies can be implemented (World Health Organization Western Pacific Region, 2012).

A strength of this project was the use of consistent methods across countries. The methods involved thorough training of research staff in data collection, which included pilot field work and reliability testing. This ensured that data were collected consistently across research teams. The food classification tool was also piloted and revised to ensure that this was relevant to each country. The study is limited by its cross-sectional design, whereby data were only captured on outdoor advertising at one point in time. Seasonal differences in advertising patterns are likely in the two study locations. Mongolia experiences extremely cold winters and so advertisements for drinks may be reduced at that time. As this study was conducted in summer, it may have overestimated the prevalence of sugar-sweetened drinks in Mongolia compared to other times of the year. In The Philippines, the study was conducted during the wet season, when extra-large billboards are dismantled to prevent their collapse onto roads and buildings. Further, massive flooding occurred in the week prior to data collection, which may have destroyed some outdoor advertisements. Therefore, the number of food advertisements observed in Manila was likely to be a conservative estimate compared to typical conditions in The Philippines.

Conclusion

This project indicates that children in Ulaanbaatar, Mongolia and Manila, The Philippines are exposed to large numbers of advertisements for unhealthy foods on their way to and from school. These advertisements are clustered within 250 m of school grounds. Notably, sugar-sweetened drinks, and particularly cola drinks, are heavily promoted near schools. These advertisements encourage the purchase and consumption of these beverages, which have been identified as a probable causal factor in weight gain and obesity. There is clear scope to reduce children's exposure to advertising for unhealthy foods in both Mongolia and The Philippines through land use and advertising regulations.

Acknowledgements

Thanks to all members of the field teams in Ulaanbaatar and Manila. Thanks also to Anthony Roda from The Philippines Department of Health and Hai-Rim Shin from the World Health Organization Regional Office for the Western Pacific.

Funding

The study was supported technically and financially by the Western Pacific Regional Office, World Health Organization. All authors confirm that they have no conflicts of interest to declare.

References

Adams, J., Ganiti, E., & White, M. (2011). Socio-economic differences in outdoor food advertising in a city in Northern England. *Public Health Nutrition, 14*, 945–950.

Cabrera Escobar, M. A., Veerman, J., Tollman, S. M., Bertram, M. Y., & Hofman, K. J. (2013). Evidence that a tax on sugar sweetened beverages reduces the obesity rate: A meta-analysis. *BMC Public Health, 13*, 1–10. doi:10.1186/1471-2458-1113-1072

Consumers International. (2008). *The junk food trap: Marketing unhealthy food to children in Asia Pacific*. Retrieved March 23, 2012, from http://www.consumersinternational.org/news-and-media/publications/junk-food-trap-a-survey-of-food-marketing-to-children-in-asia-and-the-pacific-region

Davis, B., & Carpenter, C. (2009). Proximity of fast-food restaurants to schools and adolescent obesity. *American Journal of Public Health, 99*, 505–510.

Flynn, B. C. (1996). Healthy cities: Toward worldwide health promotion. *Annual Review of Public Health, 17*, 299–309.

Hastings, G., McDermott, L., Angus, K., Stead, M., & Thomson, S. (2006). *The extent, nature and effects of food promotion to children: A review of the evidence*. Technical Paper prepared for the World Health Organization.

Hillier, A., Cole, B. L., Smith, T. E., Yancey, A. K., Williams, J. D., Grier, S. A., & McCarthy, W. J. (2009). Clustering of unhealthy outdoor advertisements around child-serving institutions: A comparison of three cities. *Health Place, 15*, 935–945.

Kamata, T., Reichert, J. A., Tsevegmid, T., Yoonhee, K., & Sedgewick, B. (2010). *Mongolia – Enhancing policies and practices for ger area development in Ulaanbaatar.* Washington, DC: World Bank.

Kelly, B., Cretikos, M., Rogers, K., & King, L. (2008). The commercial food landscape: Outdoor food advertising around primary schools in Australia. *Australian and New Zealand Journal of Public Health, 32,* 522–528.

Kelly, B., Halford, J. G. C., Boyland, E. J., Chapman, K., Bautista-Castaño, I., Berg, C., … Summerbell, C. (2010). Television food advertising to children: A global perspective. *American Journal of Public Health, 100,* 1730–1736.

Kelly, B., King, L., Chapman, K., Boyland, E., Bauman, A. E., & Baur, L. A. (in press). A hierarchy of food promotion effects: Identifying methodological approaches and knowledge gaps. *American Journal of Public Health,* Under review.

Korean Ministry of Food and Drug Safety. (2010). *The special act on the safety management of children's dietary life.* Retrieved April 17, 2013, from http://www.kfda.go.kr/eng/index.do?nMenuCode=66

Outdoor Advertising Association of the Philippines. (2006). *Code of ethics.* Retrieved January 8, 2014, from http://www.oaap.org.ph/code-of-ethics.html

Pasch, K. E., Komro, K. A., Perry, C. L., Hearst, M. O., & Farbakhsh, K. (2007). Outdoor alcohol advertising near schools: What does it advertise and how is it related to intentions and use of alcohol among young adolescents? *Journal of Studies of Alcohol and Drugs, 68,* 587–596.

Philippine Statistics Authority. (2009). *City and municipal-level small area poverty estimates.* Retrieved June 3, 2014, from http://www.nscb.gov.ph/poverty/dataCharts.asp

Stuckler, D., McKee, M., Ebrahim, S., & Basu, S. (2012). Manufacturing epidemics: The role of global producers in increased consumption of unhealthy commodities including processed foods, alcohol and tobacco. *PLOS Medicine, 9,* e1001235.

Swinburn, B., Sacks, G., Vandevijvere, S., Kumanyika, S., Lobstein, T., Neal, B., … Walker, C. (2013). INFORMAS (International Network for Food and Obesity/non-communicable diseases Research, Monitoring and Action Support): Overview and key principles. *Obesity Reviews, 14,* 1–12.

Walton, M., Pearce, J., & Day, P. (2009). Examining the interaction between food outlets and outdoor food advertisements with primary school food environments. *Health and Place, 15,* 841–848.

World Health Organization. (2003). *Diet, nutrition and the prevention of chronic diseases.* Geneva: Author.

World Health Organization. (2004). *Global strategy on diet, physical activity and health.* Geneva: Author.

World Health Organization. (2008). *School policy framework.* Retrieved January 10, 2014, from http://www.who.int/dietphysicalactivity/SPF-en-2008.pdf

World Health Organization. (2010). *Set of recommendations on the marketing of foods and non-alcoholic beverages to children.* Geneva: WHO Press.

World Health Organization. (2012). *A framework for implementing the set of recommendations on the marketing of foods and non-alcoholic beverages to children.* Geneva: WHO Press.

World Health Organization Western Pacific Region. (2012). *Japan-WHO regional consultation for promoting healthier dietary options for children (March 2012, Saitama, Japan).* Meeting Report (Report Series No. RS/2012/GE/08(JPN)). Manila: Western Pacific Regional Office, World Health Organization.

Yale Rudd Center for Food Policy and Obesity. (2013). *Pledges on food marketing to children.* Retrieved September 18, 2012, from http://www.yaleruddcenter.org/marketingpledges/search.aspx

Snack food advertising in stores around public schools in Guatemala

Violeta Chacon[a], Paola Letona[a], Eduardo Villamor[b] and Joaquin Barnoya[a,c]

[a]Department of Research, Cardiovascular Surgery Unit of Guatemala, Guatemala City, Guatemala; [b]Department of Epidemiology, University of Michigan School of Public Health, Ann Arbor, MI, USA; [c]Division of Public Health Sciences, Department of Surgery, Washington University in St. Louis, St. Louis, MO, USA

Obesity in school-age children is emerging as a public health concern. Food marketing influences preferences and increases children's requests for food. This study sought to describe the type of snack foods advertised to children in stores in and around public schools and assess if there is an association between child-oriented snack food advertising and proximity to schools. All food stores located inside and within a 200 square meter radius from two preschools and two primary schools were surveyed. We assessed store type, number, and type of snack food advertisements including those child-oriented inside and outside stores. We surveyed 55 stores and found 321 snack food advertisements. Most were on sweetened beverages (37%) and soft drinks (30%). Ninety-two (29%) were child-oriented. Atoles (100.0%), cereals (94.1%), and ice cream and frozen desserts (71.4%) had the greatest proportion of child-oriented advertising. We found more child-oriented advertisements in stores that were closer (<170 m) to schools compared with those farther away. In conclusion, the food industry is flooding the market, taking advantage of the lack of strict regulation in Guatemala. Child-oriented advertisements are available in almost all stores within a short walking distance from schools, exposing children to an obesogenic environment.

Introduction

Childhood obesity is emerging as a public health concern in Latin America (Rivera et al., 2014). Guatemala is experiencing the double burden of disease that combines a high prevalence of childhood stunting (54.5%) (World Health Organization, 2008) with a rising childhood overweight prevalence (27.1%) (World Health Organization, 2009). Overweight results from a combination of genetics, psychosocial variables, and environmental factors that affect diet and physical activity (Bouchard, 2007; Schwartz & Puhl, 2003). Among the environmental factors, food marketing is key to promote childhood weight gain (Harris, Pomeranz, Lobstein, & Brownell, 2009).

Child-oriented food marketing influences brand preferences and increases children's requests for food (Hastings et al., 2005; Letona, Chacon, Roberto, & Barnoya, 2014). Overweight and obese children have higher recognition of food advertisements and, therefore, food consumption, compared with their non-counterparts (Halford, Gillespie,

Brown, Pontin, & Dovey, 2004). A direct correlation between television advertising exposure and childhood obesity has also been documented (Gortmaker et al., 1999; Robinson, 1999). Similarly, food displays and advertisements in school kiosks are strongly associated with purchase by primary and secondary school children (Mazur et al., 2008). Furthermore, consumer segmentation, a marketing strategy that involves dividing the market into different groups with similar characteristics (e.g. age) has proven a useful tool for the food industry to increase sales (McGinnis, Appleton, & Kraak, 2006). In addition, trade liberalization policies promoting worldwide expansion of unhealthy food industry may also contribute to obesity (De Vogli, Kouvonen, & Gimeno, 2011).

In 2007, the United Kingdom was the first country to restrict television child-oriented advertising of high fat foods on all children's and non-children's channels before 9:00 PM (Ofcom, 2007). Quebec, Norway, and Sweden have also implemented bans on television food advertising and in-school marketing oriented to children (World Health Organization, 2007). Although not yet conclusive (Adams, Tyrrell, Adamson, & White, 2012), a combination of interventions, in addition to restricting television advertising, holds the most promise to decrease children's advertising exposure (Bogart, 2013; McGinnis et al., 2006). Examples include regulation of all marketing types of unhealthy foods and implementation of nutrition standards for foods and beverages sold in school kiosks (McGinnis et al., 2006).

In Guatemala, packaged foods nutrition labeling is regulated by the Food Control and Regulation Department of the Ministry of Health. According to the Department, nutrition health claims should be consistent with the nutrition information on the label (Consejo de Ministros de Integración Económica, 2012). However, to the best of our knowledge, there is no enforcement and no regulation of child-oriented food advertising (Hawkes & Lobstein, 2011). Furthermore, the types and quantity of snack foods advertised to children at the point of sale have not been documented. Moreover, the association between child-oriented snack food advertising and proximity to schools is yet unknown. Therefore, this study sought to describe the type of snack foods advertised to children in stores in and around public schools and assess if there was an association between child-oriented snack food advertising and proximity to schools.

Methods

Out of 95 public schools, two preschools and two primary schools (students between 4 and 12 years old) located in the Municipality of Mixco were conveniently selected for this study. Mixco is a city with 483,705 inhabitants (Instituto Nacional de Estadística de Guatemala, 2012) in the Department of Guatemala. Since public schools in Mixco have similar characteristics, selected schools were not likely to be atypical (Ministerio de Educación, 2012). Most children enrolled in public schools are from low socioeconomic status (World Bank, 2009) and enrollment in primary education is 95.8% (60% completion) (Guatemala Human Rights Commission Guatemala Human Rights Commission, 2010). We obtained permission from the school district supervisor and each school principal to survey kiosks inside the schools for food advertising.

All food kiosks located inside schools were surveyed. Using Google™ Earth, we identified all stores located in a 200 m radius centered on each school's entrance and surveyed the distance in meters between the school entrance and each store. We arbitrarily categorized the distance between the school entrance and stores as less than

170 m and equal or more than 170 m, as we considered this a reasonable distance for children between 4 and 12 years of age to walk to and from school.

We adapted the tobacco point of sale advertisement checklist by Cohen et al. (2008), and adapted by Barnoya, Mejia, Szeinman, and Kummerfeldt (2010) to assess the store type (i.e. small store, large store, school kiosk, street vendor, pharmacy, service station), total number of snack food advertisements, and those child-oriented inside and outside stores. We also assessed the number of stores with snack foods displayed at the counter or snack foods less than 50 cm from tobacco products, and in-store marketing techniques (display racks, refrigerators, containers, and shelves). The checklist was pilot tested in seven stores located in Mixco and found to be appropriate to assess child-oriented snack food advertisements and in-store marketing techniques. In addition, training was conducted with two research assistants one week prior to data collection.

Advertisements were defined as any posters, stickers, free-standing signs, banners, painting on walls, or flags inside or outside stores. They were considered child-oriented if they had images of promotional characters (i.e. licensed, brand-specific or sports character, cartoon, animal/creature, or celebrity), premium offers (i.e. collectibles, toys, or raffles), children's television or movie tie-ins, sports references (e.g. soccer balls, team logo), or the word "child" or synonym (e.g. junior). To allow for comparisons with previously published data (Bragg et al., 2013) on packaged snack food marketing, we included sweetened beverages (i.e. fruit and energy drinks), soft drinks, pastries and cookies, savory snacks, dairy products, cereals, ice cream and frozen desserts, and bottled water. Considering that atoles (traditional fortified cereal-based drink) are one of the most frequently consumed beverages among Guatemalan children (Montenegro-Bethancourt, Vossenaar, Doak, & Solomons, 2010), we also included packaged atoles as a category.

For data entry, we used REDCap™ web-based application. Descriptive statistics were used to summarize total and child-oriented advertisements. Median (25th–75th percentiles) was used to describe the distribution of advertisements (total, child-oriented, interior, and exterior) per store. Analyses were done with Fisher's exact and Chi-square tests for categorical variables, and Wilcoxon ranksum test for continuous variables, using STATA® software (version 11.1, 2009).

Results

We found 64 stores inside ($n = 2$) and around ($n = 62$) two preschools and two primary schools in Mixco. Nine were closed at the time of the assessment; therefore, 55 stores were surveyed. Among these were 58.2% ($n = 32$) small stores, 32.7% ($n = 18$) large stores, 5.5% ($n = 3$) street vendors, and 3.6% ($n = 2$) school kiosks. Thirteen stores (20.3%) had no advertising (six small, four large, and three street vendors).

There were 321 snack food advertisements and most were on sweetened beverages (37%) and soft drinks (30%). Twenty-eight advertisements (8.7%) were on pastries and cookies, 25 (7.8%) on savory snacks, 24 (7.5%) on dairy products, 17 (5.3%) on cereals, and 7 (2.2%) on ice cream and frozen desserts. Twenty-nine percent ($n = 92$) of all snack food advertisements found in stores were child-oriented. We found three water advertisements (no child-oriented). Atoles (100.0%), cereals (94.1%), and ice cream and frozen desserts (71.4%) had the greatest proportion of child-oriented advertising, while nine (36%) of savory snacks were child-oriented ($p < .0001$).

In stores located closer to schools (<170 m), median interior and exterior child-oriented advertisements were 1 (1–2) and 2 (1–2), respectively (Table 1). More stores located closer to schools had display racks (57.1%) and shelves (100.0%) promoting child-oriented snack foods (Table 1). In stores located farther from schools (≥170 m), we found more snack foods displayed at the counter and close (<50 cm) to tobacco products (57.1%) compared with stores closer to schools.

Discussion

In this study, we found that most advertisements in stores around schools were on sweetened beverages and soft drinks. Atoles and cereals had the greatest proportion of child-oriented advertising. Our results yield that stores closer to schools had more child-oriented advertisements compared with those farther away.

Our results are consistent with those of food advertisements around primary schools in Australia, where advertisements of unhealthy foods were higher in areas closer to schools (Kelly, Cretikos, Rogers, & King, 2008). The food industry achieves repeated brand exposure by placing advertisements in stores close to schools (Kelly et al., 2008). This has been associated with increased food consumption, and therefore higher risk of obesity (Andreyeva, Kelly, & Harris, 2011).

Age-specific market segmentation strategies are used by the food industry to reach children in schools (aged 4–12 years) and increase sales (McGinnis et al., 2006). According to our findings, one third of advertisements in stores around schools were child-oriented suggesting that the industry is using segmentation strategies to promote snack foods to children in Guatemala.

Product placement at the point-of-sale influences choice and increases sales (Glanz, Bader, & Iyer, 2012). In our sample, stores located closer to schools had more display racks and shelves promoting child-oriented snack foods, compared with those farther away. This in-store marketing technique is likely to influence children's purchase of unhealthy snacks at the point of sale. Regarding tobacco products, most stores had

Table 1. Child-oriented snack food advertising (ads) in 55 stores around four public schools in Guatemala City.

	All stores (n = 55)	<170 m from school (n = 28)	≥170 m from school (n = 27)	p*
Total ads, median (IQR)	5 (1–8)	6.5 (0–9.5)	4 (1–6)	.26
Child-oriented ads, median (IQR)	1 (0–3)	2 (0–3)	1 (0–2)	.16
Exterior child-oriented ads, median (IQR)	1 (0–2)	2 (1–2)	1 (0–2)	.11
Interior child-oriented ads, median (IQR)	1 (0–2)	1 (1–2)	.5 (0–2)	.36
Stores with interior ads that can be seen from the street, % (n)	49.1 (27)	59.3 (16)	40.7 (11)	.10
Stores with child-oriented snack foods displayed at the counter, % (n)	47.3 (26)	42.3 (11)	57.7 (15)	.89
Stores with child-oriented snack foods <50 cm from tobacco products, % (n)	12.7 (7)	42.9 (3)	57.1 (4)	.65
Stores with child-oriented in-store marketing techniques, % (n)				
Display racks	76.4 (42)	57.1 (24)	42.9 (18)	.09
Refrigerators/freezers	24.5 (14)	35.7 (5)	64.3 (9)	.19
Containers	18.2 (10)	50.0 (5)	50.0 (5)	.95
Shelves	1.8 (1)	100.0 (1)	.0 (0)	.32

*Wilcoxon rank sum test for continuous variables and Chi-square test for categorical variables.

tobacco products displayed near snack foods. Therefore, as tobacco, the food industry is using the point of sale as yet unregulated marketing strategy in Guatemala. Placing both products is associated with increased brand recognition and consumption (or initiation in the case of cigarettes) (Barnoya et al., 2010; Henriksen, Schleicher, Feighery, & Fortmann, 2010; Hosler & Kammer, 2012).

Snack food advertising has been previously documented near schools and in neighborhoods of different socioeconomic status in different countries (Batada, Seitz, Wootan, & Story, 2008; Gebauer & Laska, 2011; Maher, Wilson, & Signal, 2005). Unhealthy snack food and beverage advertising has been found to be higher in stores (including near schools) and in low socioeconomic status neighborhoods (Yancey et al., 2009). However, only one has focused on child-oriented advertising and distance from school, and included all advertising (Kelly et al., 2008). Our findings are in agreement with what has been previously published and add that child-oriented snack food advertising is highly prevalent near schools in Guatemala, a LMIC.

Even though data on the companies responsible for advertising snack foods in Guatemala is lacking, multinational companies (e.g. PepsiCo, The Coca-Cola Company) dominate the beverage market as in the rest of Latin America (Comision Economica para América Latina y el Caribe, 2005). Therefore, globalization is disproportionately benefiting multinational companies, promoting economic inequality, and fueling the obesity epidemic (De Vogli, Kouvonen, Elovainio, & Marmot, 2013).

Our study should be viewed in light of some limitations. We only described child-oriented snack food advertisements and not all food advertisements. Similar to the Bragg, et al. study (Bragg et al., 2013), advertising of confectioneries were not included, and therefore our results cannot be generalized to these snacks also marketed to children. Additionally, even though our sample was not intended to be representative of the entire country, child-oriented advertisements are likely to be the same nationwide considering convenience stores are found in almost every neighborhood nationwide.

In conclusion, child-oriented snack food advertising at the point of sale is a strategy widely used by the food industry to reach children. Just as the tobacco industry takes advantage of the unregulated environment in Guatemala, point of sale advertising is only one of several channels the food industry uses. Any effort to promote healthy eating inside schools would be ruled out by the heavy exposure to this pervasive form of marketing in stores around schools. Therefore, any comprehensive population strategy aiming to decrease exposure to unhealthy snack food advertising should include the point of sale just as other traditional advertising venues. While the food industry would likely oppose, a ban on snack food advertisements in stores around schools is possible, similar to tobacco advertising restrictions.

Funding

This work was carried out with the aid of a grant from the International Development Research Centre, Ottawa, Canada [Project number 106883-001]. Joaquin Barnoya receives additional support from an unrestricted grant from the American Cancer Society and from Barnes Jewish Hospital Foundation. Additional support was received from NIH Research Grant [# D43 TW009315] funded by the Fogarty International Center.

Supplemental data

Supplemental data for this article can be accessed here: http://dx.doi.org/10.1080/09581596.2014.953035.

References

Adams, J., Tyrrell, R., Adamson, A. J., & White, M. (2012). Effect of restrictions on television food advertising to children on exposure to advertisements for 'less healthy' foods: Repeat cross-sectional study. *PLoS ONE, 7*, e31578. doi:10.1371/journal.pone.0031578PONE-D-11-21779 [pii]

Andreyeva, T., Kelly, I. R., & Harris, J. L. (2011). Exposure to food advertising on television: Associations with children's fast food and soft drink consumption and obesity. *Economics & Human Biology, 9*, 221–233. doi:10.1016/j.ehb.2011.02.004S1570-677X(11)00029-3 [pii]

Barnoya, J., Mejia, R., Szeinman, D., & Kummerfeldt, C. E. (2010). Tobacco point-of-sale advertising in Guatemala City, Guatemala and Buenos Aires, Argentina. *Tobacco Control, 19*, 338–341. doi:10.1136/tc.2009.031898tc.2009.031898 [pii]

Batada, A., Seitz, M. D., Wootan, M. G., & Story, M. (2008). Nine out of 10 food advertisements shown during Saturday morning children's television programming are for foods high in fat, sodium, or added sugars, or low in nutrients. *Journal of the American Dietetic Association, 108*, 673–678. doi:10.1016/j.jada.2008.01.015 [pii]

Bogart, W. A. (2013). Law as a tool in "the war on obesity": Useful interventions, maybe, but, first, what's the problem? *Journal of Law, Medicine and Ethics, 41*, 28–41. doi:10.1111/jlme.12003

Bouchard, C. (2007). The biological predisposition to obesity: Beyond the thrifty genotype scenario. *International Journal of Obesity, 31*, 1337–1339. doi:10.1038/sj.ijo.0803610

Bragg, M. A., Liu, P. J., Roberto, C. A., Sarda, V., Harris, J. L., & Brownell, K. D. (2013). The use of sports references in marketing of food and beverage products in supermarkets. *Public Health Nutrition, 16*, 738–742. doi:10.1017/S1368980012003163 [pii]

Chapman, K., Nicholas, P., Banovic, D., & Supramaniam, R. (2006). The extent and nature of food promotion directed to children in Australian supermarkets. *Health Promotion International, 21*, 331–339. doi:10.1093/heapro/dal028 [pii]

Cohen, J. E., Planinac, L. C., Griffin, K., Robinson, D. J., O'Connor, S. C., Lavack, A., ... Di Nardo, J. (2008). Tobacco promotions at point-of-sale: The last hurrah. *Canadian Journal of Public Health, 99*, 166–171.

Comision Economica para América Latina y el Caribe. (2005). *Las translatinas en la industria de los alimentos y bebidas.* Retrieved from http://www.cepal.org/publicaciones/xml/4/24294/lcg2309e_Cap_V.pdf

Consejo de Ministros de Integración Económica. (2012). *Reglamento técnico centroamericano del etiquetado de productos alimenticios preenvasados para consumo humano para la población a partir de 3 años de edad.* Retrieved from http://www.dgrs.gob.hn/documents/Resoluciones/AlimentosBebidas/17990000004172RTCAEtiqNutricional.pdf

De Vogli, R., Kouvonen, A., Elovainio, M., & Marmot, M. (2013). Economic globalization, inequality and body mass index: A cross-national analysis of 127 countries. *Critical Public Health, 24*, 7–21.

De Vogli, R., Kouvonen, A., & Gimeno, D. (2011). "Globesization": Ecological evidence on the relationship between fast food outlets and obesity among 26 advanced economies. *Critical Public Health, 21*, 395–402.

Dixon, H., Scully, M., & Parkinson, K. (2006). Pester power: Snackfoods displayed at supermarket checkouts in Melbourne, Australia. *Health Promotion Journal of Australia, 17*, 124–127.

Gebauer, H., & Laska, M. N. (2011). Convenience stores surrounding urban schools: An assessment of healthy food availability, advertising, and product placement. *Journal of Urban Health, 88*, 616–622. doi:10.1007/s11524-011-9576-3

Glanz, K., Bader, M. D., & Iyer, S. (2012). Retail grocery store marketing strategies and obesity. *American Journal of Preventive Medicine, 42*, 503–512. doi:10.1016/j.amepre.2012.01. 013S0749-3797(12)00058-X [pii]

Gortmaker, S. L., Peterson, K., Wiecha, J., Sobol, A. M., Dixit, S., Fox, M. K., & Laird, N. (1999). Reducing obesity via a school-based interdisciplinary intervention among youth. *Archives of Pediatrics and Adolescent Medicine, 153*, 409–418.

Grigsby-Toussaint, D. S., Moise, I. K., & Geiger, S. D. (2011). Observations of marketing on food packaging targeted to youth in retail food stores. *Obesity, 19*, 1898–1900. doi:10.1038/ oby.2011.120 [pii]

Guatemala Human Rights Commission. 2010. *Education in Guatemala Fact Sheet.* Retrieved from http://www.ghrc-usa.org/Publications/factsheet_education.pdf

Halford, J. C., Gillespie, J., Brown, V., Pontin, E. E., & Dovey, T. M. (2004). Effect of television advertisements for foods on food consumption in children. *Appetite, 42*, 221–225. doi:10.1016/j.appet.2003.11.006S0195666303001910 [pii]

Harris, J. L., Pomeranz, J. L., Lobstein, T., & Brownell, K. D. (2009). A crisis in the market-place: How food marketing contributes to childhood obesity and what can be done. *Annual Review of Public Health, 30*, 211–225. doi:10.1146/annurev.publhealth.031308.100304

Hastings, G., Stead, M., McDermott, L., Forsyth, A., MacKintosh, A., Rayner, M., … Angus, K. (2005). *The extent, nature and effects of food promotion to children: A review of the evidence.* Retrieved from http://libdoc.who.int/publications/2007/9789241595247_eng.pdf

Hawkes, C., & Lobstein, T. (2011). Regulating the commercial promotion of food to children: A survey of actions worldwide. *International Journal of Pediatric Obesity, 6*, 83–94. doi:10.3109/17477166.2010.486836

Henriksen, L., Schleicher, N. C., Feighery, E. C., & Fortmann, S. P. (2010). A longitudinal study of exposure to retail cigarette advertising and smoking initiation. *Pediatrics, 126*, 232–238. doi:10.1542/peds.2009-3021peds.2009-3021 [pii]

Hosler, A. S., & Kammer, J. R. (2012). Point-of-purchase tobacco access and advertisement in food stores. *Tobacco Control, 21*, 451–452. doi:10.1136/tobaccocontrol-2011-050221tobacco-control-2011-050221 [pii]

Instituto Nacional de Estadística de Guatemala. 2012. *Estimaciones de la Población Total por Municipio.* Retrieved from http://www.ine.gob.gt/

Kelly, B., Cretikos, M., Rogers, K., & King, L. (2008). The commercial food landscape: Outdoor food advertising around primary schools in Australia. *Australian and New Zealand Journal of Public Health, 32*, 522–528. doi:10.1111/j.1753-6405.2008.00303.xAZPH303 [pii]

Letona, P., Chacon, V., Roberto, C., & Barnoya, J. (2014). Effects of licensed characters on chil-dren's taste and snack preferences in Guatemala, a low/middle income country. *International Journal of Pediatric Obesity (Lond).* doi:10.1038/ijo.2014.38

Maher, A., Wilson, N., & Signal, L. (2005). Advertising and availability of 'obesogenic' foods around New Zealand secondary schools: A pilot study. *New Zealand Medical Journal, 118*, 10–20.

Mazur, A., Telega, G., Kotowicz, A., Malek, H., Jarochowicz, S., Gierczak, B., … Mazur, D. (2008). Impact of food advertising on food purchases by students in primary and secondary schools in south-eastern Poland. *Public Health Nutrition, 11*, 978–981. doi:10.1017/ S1368980008002000S1368980008002000 [pii]

McGinnis, J. M., Appleton, J., & Kraak, V. (2006). *Food marketing to children and youth: Threat or opportunity?* Washington, DC: The National Academies Press.

Montenegro-Bethancourt, G., Vossenaar, M., Doak, C. M., & Solomons, N. W. (2010). Contribu-tion of beverages to energy, macronutrient and micronutrient intake of third- and fourth-grade schoolchildren in Quetzaltenango, Guatemala. *Maternal and Child Nutrition, 6*, 174–189. doi:10.1111/j.1740-8709.2009.00193.xMCN193 [pii]

Ofcom. 2007. *Television advertising of food and drink products to children. Final statement.* Retrieved from http://stakeholders.ofcom.org.uk/binaries/consultations/foodads_new/statement/ statement.pdf

Probart, C., McDonnell, E., Bailey-Davis, L., & Weirich, J. E. (2006). Existence and predictors of soft drink advertisements in Pennsylvania high schools. *Journal of the American Dietetic Association, 106*, 2052–2056. doi:10.1016/j.jada.2006.09.013 [pii]

Rivera, J. A., Cossio, T., Pedraza, L., Aburto, T., Sanchez, T., & Martorell, R. (2014). Childhood and adolescent overweight and obesity in Latin America: A systematic review. *The Lancet Diabetes & Endocrinology, 2*, 321–332. doi:10.1016/S2213-8587(13)70173-6

Robinson, T. N. (1999). Reducing children's television viewing to prevent obesity. *JAMA, 282*, 1561–1567. doi:joc90434 [pii]

Schwartz, M. B., & Puhl, R. (2003). Childhood obesity: A societal problem to solve. *Obesity Reviews, 4*, 57–71.

Walton, M., Pearce, J., & Day, P. (2009). Examining the interaction between food outlets and outdoor food advertisements with primary school food environments. *Health & Place, 15*, 811–848. doi:10.1016/j.healthplace.2009.02.003 [pii]

World Bank. 2009. *Guatemala poverty assessment good performance at low levels.* Retrieved from http://siteresources.worldbank.org/INTLACREGTOPPOVANA/Resources/GuatemalaPov ertyAssessmentEnglish.pdf

World Health Organization. 2007. *Marketing food to children: Changes in the global regulatory environment 2004–2006.* Retrieved from http://www.who.int/dietphysicalactivity/regula tory_environment_CHawkes07.pdf

World Health Organization. 2008. *Malnutrition in infants and young children in Latin America and the Caribbean: Achieving the millennium development goals.* Retrieved from http://www. unscn.org/layout/modules/resources/files/Malnutrition_in_Infants_and_Young_Children_in_ LAC,__Achieving_the_MDGs.pdf

World Health Organization. 2009. *Guatemala global school-based student health survey.* Retrieved from http://www.who.int/chp/gshs/2009_Guatemala_GSHS_Questionnaire.pdf

Ministerio de Educación. (2012). *Anuario Estadístico.* Retrieved from http://www.mineduc.gob.gt/ estadistica/2012/main.html

Yancey, A. K., Cole, B. L., Brown, R., Williams, J. D., Hillier, A., Kline, R. S., … McCarthy, W. J. (2009). A cross-sectional prevalence study of ethnically targeted and general audience outdoor obesity-related advertising. *Milbank Quarterly, 87*, 155–184. doi:10.1111/j.1468-0009.2009.00551.xMILQ551 [pii]

The incursion of 'Big Food' in middle-income countries: a qualitative documentary case study analysis of the soft drinks industry in China and India

Simon N. Williams

Feinberg School of Medicine, Northwestern University, Chicago, IL, USA

Public health research is only just beginning to explore the myriad ways in which the food and beverage industry, or 'Big Food', has sought to influence policy and increase consumption of energy-dense products high in sugar, salt, and fat in middle-income countries. In particular, very little research has focused on Asia-Pacific markets, including China and India. This article uses the soft drink sector as a case study, and focuses on The Coca-Cola Company – the largest soft drinks company in both China and India. Documentary data from company reports, news articles, industry analyst reports, and industry magazines are analyzed to explore how the company successfully re-entered these markets following liberalization of their economies, and how it subsequently sought to influence government and key organizations in order to increase consumption and challenge public health policy. Applying a framework previously used in an analysis of Big Food in high income countries like the United States, I find that Coca-Cola has used the same strategies in China and India. Findings reveal that Coca-Cola lobbied US Government officials (in order to influence international issues); made political contributions; participated in a 'revolving door' between government and industry; funded professional organizations; and generally lobbied to resist regulation or urge weak regulation. The findings of this study could help to inform public health debates about Big Food in other emerging markets, including the Middle East and Africa.

Over the past decade, public health research has begun to explore the myriad ways in which the food and beverage industry, or 'Big Food', has sought to influence policy and increase consumption of energy-dense products high in sugar, salt, and fat in high-income countries (HICs) like the United States (Nestle, 2002; Stuckler & Nestle, 2012). However, Big Food's role in the 'westernization' (Pingali, 2007) of middle-income countries (MICs) – what Popkin (2012) terms the 'nutrition transition' – is only beginning to receive due attention (Basu, 2015; Chacon, Letona, Villamor, & Barnoya, 2015; Igumbor et al., 2012; Kelly et al., 2015; Monteiro & Cannon, 2012). Very little in-depth attention has been paid to Big Food's influence in the Asia-Pacific markets, including China and India. Big Food companies have explicitly stated their intent to focus on MICs (PepsiCo, 2011; Nestlé, 2011). Coca-Cola, for example, has invested $4 billion in

China over the past two years (Coca-Cola, 2013) and plans to invest $5 billion in India by 2020 (Gulati & Ahmed, 2012). It is essential, therefore, that public health research explores this issue before this incursion gets deeper still.

According to Brownell and Warner (2009), one of the main strategies through which Big Food has shaped public policy and increased the consumption of unhealthy foods and beverages in the United States is by influencing government and key organizations. This influence, along with strategies for public relations and framing, disputing science and 'creating doubt', and product marketing, comprises Big Food's 'corporate play-book'; a playbook which Brownell and Warner (2009) liken to that of the tobacco industry. Brownell and Warner (2009) discuss how companies influence government and key organizations through a number of activities, including *lobbying US Government officials* (in order to influence international issues); *making political contributions*; *participating in a 'revolving door' between government and industry*; *funding professional organizations*; and generally *lobbying to resist regulation or urge weak regulation*. Brownell and Warner (2009) argue that whereas the industry needs to take more responsibility for rising obesity rates – instead of emphasizing that obesity is a personal responsibility – political agencies also have a responsibility to avoid being 'captured' by industry.

In this article, I examine the 'transferability' (Guba, 1981) of Brownell and Warner's (2009) analysis of Big Food's strategies to influence government and key organizations to two MICs – China and India. I ask whether, to what extent, and in what ways, a multinational Big Food company has influenced government and key organizations in order to shape public policy and increase product consumption in these two countries. In so doing, I also discuss some novel challenges specific to emerging markets, including navigating the potential barriers to market entry. This article focuses on the Coca-Cola Company (hereafter Coca-Cola) – the 'world's most powerful brand' (Ani, 2014), the world's largest soft drink company, and currently, the largest soft drinks company in both countries (Euromonitor International, 2013).

Methods

Grounded in similar research on other industries, particularly the tobacco industry, (e.g. Smith, Fooks, Collin, Weishaar, & Gilmore, 2010; also Gilmore, 2005; Shirane et al., 2012), this paper takes a public health perspective in critically interpreting documents that focus on the activities of the Coca-Cola Company in China and India. Specifically, this paper is set within a critical tradition of corporatology that seeks to analyze industries and multinational companies in certain sectors selling 'unhealthy commodities' (Stuckler, McKee, Ebrahim, & Basu, 2012) (e.g. tobacco, alcohol, sugar-sweetened soft drinks and 'junk' food) as potential 'vectors of disease' (Guardino & Daynard, 2007; Jahiel, 2008; Jahiel & Babor, 2007; Orleans & Slade, 1993). Thus, in terms of reflexivity, it is important to acknowledge that this critical perspective informs the interpretation of the documents analyzed, and thus the findings of this paper.

Data for this study were taken from the following documentary sources: company annual and quarterly reports; market reports; news media articles; and food and beverage industry magazines and journals. Coca-Cola annual and quarterly reports (2003–2014) were downloaded from the company's website and analyzed in detail. Newspaper articles (including all English language publications) were found using Nexis database searches. Building on a methodology well-established in tobacco industry research (Gilmore, 2005), documents were identified using a structured but iterative search, and were assessed for relevance. The date range was fixed at 1975–2012 – to cover the company's activity during the liberalization of the Indian and Chinese markets. The following keywords were used to guide the search: 'China', 'Chinese', 'India', 'Indian', and 'Coca-Cola' or 'Coke'. Articles were deemed relevant if they had as their primary focus the Coca-Cola Company and its activities in China or India, or issues that pertained to China or India. A total of 429 newspaper articles were identified and reviewed. To supplement these articles, search engine searches of online news articles were conducted for articles published between 2012 and 2014. Additionally, 208 industry magazine articles were analyzed in depth. Back issues and/or news archives of the following industry magazines were searched and examined for articles relating to China and India: Soft Drinks International (June 2009–February 2011), Beverage Daily (April 2002–June 2012), Just Drinks (May 2000–Jun 2012), and Bevnet (formerly Beverage Spectrum) (Nov/Dec 2007–June 2012). Finally, market reports ($n = 7$) were primarily drawn from EuroMonitor Passport Global Market Information database. Reports pertaining to soft drinks, the Coca-Cola Company in China and India as well as to global strategy were consulted.

Documents were interpreted using an approach established within tobacco industry research (Gilmore, 2005; Lee & Collin, 2006), wherein documents were triangulated across sources in order to reconstruct a narrative of events and explore company activities, informed by the critical perspective discussed above. All documents were analyzed using a framework approach (Ritchie & Spencer, 2002), which is a thematic approach to analysis. Qualitative data are coded and organized according to themes and subthemes, allowing for the incorporation of both a priori themes and those that emerge inductively through the analytical process. This approach entailed five key methodological stages: familiarization; identifying a thematic framework; indexing; charting; mapping and interpretation (Ritchie & Spencer, 2002). In this study, all these stages were addressed. Brief reviews of the documents allowed familiarization with the overall topic. This was particularly important in the absence of extensive academic literature on Big Food in MICs. Before documents not directly relevant to the study's aims could be excluded, a thematic framework was necessary. Following the brief review, provisional notes were made on prominent and recurring themes that related to the ways in which Coca-Cola sought to influence government and key organizations. Themes were derived a priori from Brownell and Warner's (2009) analysis, and inductively from the data as they began to emerge. The documentary themes were displayed in data matrices that provided an overview of the analysis. One function of the analysis was to assess the 'transferability' of Brownell and Warner's (2009) framework of Big Food strategies to influence government and key organizations. Guba (1981) defines transferability as 'the degree of similarity (fittingness) between two contexts'. Shenton (2004) notes that the accumulation of findings from studies staged in different settings might enable a more inclusive, overall picture to be gained. Thus, in trying to fully understand the global practices of Big Food companies, the analysis of multiple national contexts is beneficial. The analysis in this study sought to examine whether existing knowledge on the strategies that companies have employed in HICs – captured in Brownell and Warner's (2009) framework – are similar to or different from the strategies they have employed in MICs. Also, as will be discussed below, this detailed analysis of the Chinese and Indian cases also serves as an empirical grounding for future analyses of other MICs and emerging markets.

The growth of the soft drink market in China and India

Within the medical and public health communities, it is widely acknowledged that increases in the consumption of free sugar had made a substantial contribution to the growing rates of obesity and diabetes in a number of countries worldwide. Obesity is a complex public health problem and it is important to note that soft drinks are of course not solely responsible for the increase in obesity and diabetes rates in China and India. Recent draft guidelines from the World Health Organization (WHO) have recommended that intake of free sugars is reduced and that free sugars should account for less than 10% of total daily energy. The guidelines were based on a systematic review and meta-analysis, commissioned by the WHO, which concluded that increased sugar intake was associated with increased body weight, and that sugar-sweetened beverage intake was associated with higher body weight in children (Briggs, 2014; Lobstein, 2014; WHO, 2014). Additionally, recent epidemiological studies have shown how soft drinks are significantly associated with rising overweight, obesity, and diabetes prevalence, both globally and specifically in low- and middle-income countries like China and India (Basu, McKee, Galea, & Stuckler, 2013).

It is also important to acknowledge that the overall market category 'soft drinks' does include some products, like bottled water, that aren't an unhealthy commodity. However, carbonates and energy/sports drinks (many of which are sugar-sweetened) still make up more than a third of the global soft drinks market (approximately 175 billion liters out of 465 billion liters in 2011) (Euromonitor International, 2013). Moreover, while in the US, total energy per capita and average energy density of beverages sold has decreased; in China, the opposite is true (Kleiman, Ng, & Popkin, 2012). Relatedly, although diet carbonates are popular in HICs (in the United States, diet colas account for one-third of all cola carbonates), they are far less popular and available in India (Taylor, Satija, Khurana, Singh, & Ebrahim, 2010), where they remain a 'niche drink' accounting for less than 2% of cola carbonates volume sales (Euromonitor International, 2005, 2011).

One of the barriers to the substitution of diet beverages for sugar-sweetened beverages is that Big Food does not want their diet colas to 'cannibalize' the market share of their sugar-sweetened colas. A recent industry analyst's report noted that Coca-Cola 'must continue to sustain growth in standard cola and expand low calorie cola' (Euromonitor, 2013). Table 1 shows how overall, in China and India, Coca-Cola and its major rival PepsiCo have a far greater share of the carbonates markets relative to their share of the bottled water or juice markets. At the same time as Coca-Cola increasingly focuses its efforts on India's rural markets (Euromonitor, 2013) – which consist of more than 70% of the total population – rates of obesity and overweight are starting to rise in these areas. This is particularly concerning, given that rural populations are still vastly underserved by health care when compared to urban areas (Balarajan, Selvaraj, & Subramanian, 2011). In China, Coca-Cola is the market leader with a total market share of 14.3% (compared to nearest rival PepsiCo's share of 4.5%) (Euromonitor International, 2013). Coca-Cola is also the market leader in India, with a total market share of 23.3% (compared to that of domestic company Parle Biserli at 22.8% and PepsiCo's at 20.9%) (Table 1).

There have been sharp increases in per capita consumption of soft drinks in China and India since the late 1990s, at the same time as the percentage of the average daily disposable income required to purchase soft drinks has decreased (Figures 1 and 2).

In China, annual per capita soft drink consumption by 2016 is predicted to be more than 10 times (76.8 L) higher than it was in 1997 (7.4 L). In India, per capita soft drink

Table 1. Percentage of soft drink market shares (total and by category) of Coca-Cola and Pepsi-Co in China and India.

Market shares (2013)	Company	
	The Coca-Cola company	Pepsi-Co
China		
% Market share – total soft drinks	14.3	4.5
% Market share – carbonates	62.1	29.2
% Market share – sports and energy drinks	NA/unavailable	4.8
% Market share – bottled water	6.0	NA/unavailable
% Market share – juice	12.7	1.2
India		
% Market share – total soft drinks	23.3	20.9
% Market share – carbonates	59.6	35.5
% Market share – sports and energy drinks	0.9	34.9
% Market share – bottled water	10.5	15.3
% Market share – juice	31.4	27.6

Note: Figures taken from Euromonitor International (2013) Data-set: Soft Drinks (www.portal.eu romonitor.com).

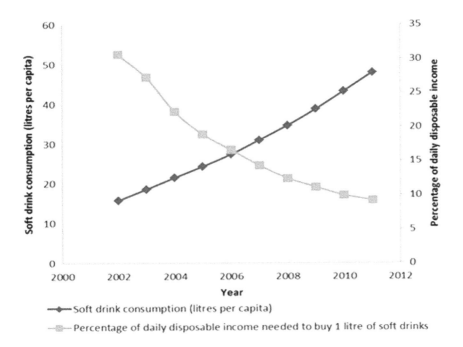

Figure 1. Per capita soft drink consumption vs. percentage of daily disposable income required to buy 1 L of soft drinks, China 2002–2011.

consumption by 2016 is predicted to be 13 times (15.7 L) higher than it was in 1997 (1.2 L) (Euromonitor International, 2013). These two markets are particularly appealing to Coca-Cola precisely because they still have considerable room for growth, unlike the established HIC markets – where per capita consumption has plateaued. In a recent

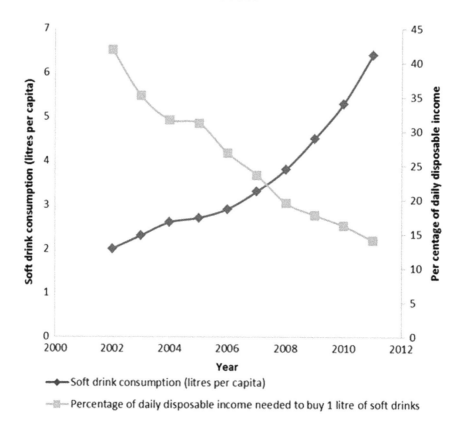

Figure 2. Per capita soft drink consumption vs. percentage of daily disposable income required to buy 1 L of soft drinks, India 2002–2011.

report, an industry analyst concluded that if per capita consumption in China was comparable to that of the United States, then the market would be worth US$717.5 billion, four times that of the US soft drinks market (in 2009) (Euromonitor, 2010). Figures from 2012 show how total annual off-trade volume sales in China have nearly matched those in the US (approximately 71 billion liters compared to approximately 79 billion liters), and are due to surpass them by the end of 2014 (Euromonitor International, 2013). Should the Chinese spend and drink like Americans (Euromonitor International, 2010), this will fulfill a 20-year-old ambition of former Coca-Cola CEO Roberto Goizueta to 'increase Chinese consumption of Coca-Cola drinks to that in the United States' (Janofsky, 1993).

Navigating political barriers to entry in new markets: how Coca-Cola pioneered in China, but followed in India

As has been the case in research on the tobacco industry (Gilmore, 2005), an analysis of multinational companies' market entry strategies can help shed light on how they utilize existing international political connections and on how they establish new domestic political connections. Because the political and market structures in MICs are often different to those in HICs, entering new food and beverage markets in MICs can be particularly challenging for Big Food. Central to a multinational company's success in a new market is the timing of its entry and the strategies they use to enter. Lilien and Yoon (1990) propose two main strategies for companies when entering new markets: pioneering and following. Coca-Cola's paths to becoming the biggest multinational soft drink company in China and India differed between the two countries. Whilst they pioneered the Chinese soft drink market, in India, they followed their major competitor, PepsiCo. Both modes of market entry entail risks and benefits. Whereas the pioneer sees the potential advantages of building reputation and profit advantage, they also have the potential disadvantages of absorbing the risks and costs associated with product and market development (Lilien & Yoon, 1990). However, Coca-Cola has shown how each can be used as a means through which to capture the leading share of an emerging market.

Coca-Cola first entered China in the 1920s, but was effectively forced out of the country as a result of the Mao era of Communism during the 1950s (Pendergrast, 2000). The company did, however, become the first American company to import and sell their products in China after trade relations between the two countries were normalized in 1979 (Kleinfield, 1978). Although denied by the company, close personal links between US President Carter and Coca-Cola Chairman and Chief Executive, J. Paul Austin, were claimed to be instrumental in facilitating the company's re-entry into the Chinese market (Eichenwald, 1985; Jensen, 1978; Kleinfield, 1978). The company worked hard during the 1970s to increase its acceptance in China, by sponsoring numerous cultural events and sporting teams, offering Harvard scholarships to Chinese students (Koten, 1980; Sterba, 1981; Washington Post, 1979), and cultivating political ties with high-profile Chinese politicians, including the then Deputy Prime Minister Teng Hsiao-ping (Butterfield, 1979; McNulty, 1979). Despite tight market restrictions, Coca-Cola's distribution and sales grew significantly during the 1980s, aided by a series of joint ventures with the Chinese Government (Janofsky, 1993), and a number of strategic partnerships with foreign groups, like Hong Kong's Kerry and Swire bottling companies, who had 'strong political connections to the Chinese Government' (Mok, Dai, & Yeung, 2002; Weisert, 2001). Coca-Cola was therefore at the forefront of the expansion of the soft drinks industry, where the total number of soft drink plants across all companies rose considerably from 130 in 1981 to at least 2700 in 1991 (Nolan, 1996).

In India, Coca-Cola was forced to adopt a different strategy in order to establish itself as the soft drinks market leader. Although Coke had first been available since the early 1950s, a dispute with the Indian Government, in which it refused to reveal its product's ingredients and reduce its equity as part of the Foreign Exchange Regulation Act (FERA), meant that the company had to withdraw from the country in 1977 (Chicago Tribune, 1977; Rangan, 1977; NY Times, 1977). Against this background, the company sought more independence in their re-entry, but had a $3 million bid to build a plant in the country rejected by the Indian Government (NY Times, 1990). This allowed the company's main rival PepsiCo to capitalize on their $17 million agreement with the Indian Government in 1990, following 'half a decade of negotiating, 20 debates in Parliament and a monumental public relations campaign' (Crossette, 1990). During entry, PepsiCo was criticized for capitalizing on the political and economic unrest in the troubled northern state of Punjab (Weisman, 1988). The company was also criticized for using their food processing side-venture and their stated focus on exports as a 'ruse' for their real aim of breaking the domestic soft drinks market (Weisman, 1988). However, if PepsiCo used these strategies 'to enter the Indian market through the back door' (Barnetson, 1986), then by the time they finally entered in 1993,

Coca-Cola was able to walk in straight through the front door of a market which was by now more favorable to foreign investment. Rather than focusing on building the local brand equity of its own international products, Coca-Cola acquired an instant majority market share. From domestic company Parle, it bought five of India's top-selling domestic brands, including the biggest domestic cola brand 'Thums Up'. By the end of 1993, the company had acquired more than 60% of the Indian soft drinks market (Gulati & Ahmed, 2012). Although Coca-Cola's market share has since been reduced, sustained heavy investment in India, to a total of US$2 billion (Coca-Cola, 2012a), has ensured that it has remained the market leader (Euromonitor International, 2013).

Coca-Cola was able to pioneer in China because it had cultivated good political relations, thus enabling them to use joint ventures, a lower risk strategy in unfamiliar markets, as their primary market entry mode. In India, because of weaker political relations, Coca-Cola initially followed behind market pioneer PepsiCo. Because PepsiCo had already successfully tested the Indian market by the time Coca-Cola re-entered, the latter was able to minimize the risks normally associated with large acquisitions of domestic brands and facilities in new markets.

Influencing government and key organizations

As noted above, Big Food's strategies to influence government and key organizations in the United States include: *lobbying US Government officials* (in order to influence international issues); *making political contributions*; *participating in a 'revolving door' between government and industry*; *funding professional organizations*; and generally *lobbying to resist regulation or urge weak regulation* (Brownell & Warner, 2009). As the case of Coca-Cola in China and India attests, we see the same strategies being used to influence government and key organizations in MICs.

Lobbying US Government officials

The US–China Business Council (USCBC) and the US–India Business Council (USIBC) are examples of vehicles through which Big Food can seek to influence trade policies in China and India, in order to make them more favorable to growth and investment. For example, the USCBC has lobbied in favor of reducing tariffs and other market access barriers on foods produced outside China (USCBC, 2012a). Events hosted by such councils create opportunities for senior figures from the food and drink industry to engage senior political figures, both from the United States and from China or India. Between 2010 and 2012, Coca-Cola CEO Muktar Kent was Chair of a USCBC Board that also included PepsiCo's CEO Indra Nooyi (USCBC, 2010). During this time, the USCBC co-hosted a roundtable between industry CEOs and senior American and Chinese political figures, including US Vice-President Joe Biden and Chinese Vice-President Xi Jinping, during the latter's visit to the United States. Also, during Jinping's visit, Kent addressed a group of 'nearly 600 corporate and policy leaders', including former Secretary of State Henry Kissinger and then Commerce Secretary John Bryson (China Business Review, 2011; Kellerhals, 2012). Coca-Cola have also sponsored USCBC events, where US and Chinese Government officials, including China's Ambassador to the United States, joined business leaders in order to discuss bilateral commercial relations between the countries (China Business Review, 2010b).

Making political contributions

Through its 'political action committees' (PACs), Coca-Cola has made political contributions to American politicians who play important roles in governmental groups focused on relations between the United States and China or India.

The USCBC has hosted annual receptions for the US–China Working Group in the House of Representatives (China Business Review, 2010a). One of the aims of the US–China Working Group is to 'educate' members of Congress on US–China issues (Larsen, 2013). As noted above, UCSBC events provide opportunities for senior representatives from the food and beverage industry to engage senior political figures, including Senators Harry Reid and Mitch McConnell (Kellerhals, 2012). Reid and McConnell, along with the founders of the US–China Working Group in the House of Representatives – Senators Rick Larsen and Mark Kirk – have received political donations (a combined total of $27,500) from Coca-Cola's Political Action Committee (PAC) between 2007 and 2011 (Coca-Cola, 2007, 2008, 2009, 2011).

The US Senate's India Caucus was established as a forum for senators to work closely with Indian Government officials in promoting US–India relations. Across 2012 and 2013, Coca-Cola's PACs have made financial campaign contributions to two-thirds of the membership (28 out of 42 members) of the Senate's India Caucus, amounting to a total of $104,000 (including $9000 to its co-founder and current co-chair, Senator John Cornyn) (Coca-Cola, 2012b, 2013).

Participating in the 'revolving door'

The 'revolving door' phenomenon is where regulators tend to be more supportive of an industry when they have a background in that industry or when they expect rewards in the form of future employment in that industry (Cohen, 1986; Makkai & Braithwaite, 1992). In instances where former regulators move into industry positions, they bring 'lobbying capital' in the form of their political contacts (Dal Bo, 2006). Brownell and Warner (2009) discuss how the US Department of Agriculture (USDA) was prone to 'regulatory capture' because many of its leaders would be recruited from, and then return to, the food and agriculture industry. In India, there is evidence that Coca-Cola has participated in a revolving door with government. Most notably, Arun Jaitley, currently serving as Minister of Finance, Minister of Defence, and Minister of Corporate Affairs, and referred to as 'the most important person in the new government after Prime Minister Narendra Modi' (IndiaToday, 2014), has previously worked as a lawyer defending both Coca-Cola and PepsiCo (Sahu & Kala, 2014). Also, at least half of the members of Coca-Cola India's Advisory Board have previously occupied at least one government position (Businessweek, 2014). Strong prior associations with the financial, economic, and trade departments and agencies in the Indian Government are particularly evident. For example, Nand Singh's government positions included serving as 'the main Economic Advisor to the Prime Minister, in charge of overall macro-economic policies, medium term economic strategy and infrastructure at Central and State Government' (Businessweek, 2014). Sunil Munjal served in numerous positions, including as a member of the Prime Minister's Council on Trade and Industry and as a committee member of the Ministry of Finance and Company Affairs' Task Force on Indirect Taxes (Businessweek, 2014). Naresh Chandra, with stated expertise in economic reforms, has occupied a number of high-profile political positions, including Senior Adviser to the Prime Minister and Indian Ambassador to the United States (Businessweek, 2014).

Funding professional organizations

Brownell and Warner (2009) note how Big Food fund and use major lobbying vehicles to influence policy at the state, national, and international levels. The International Life Sciences Institute (ILSI) is a corporate lobby group founded in 1978 by Coca-Cola and PepsiCo, General Foods, Kraft and Proctor & Gamble, and was led until 1991 by Coca-Cola Vice-President Alex Malaspina (Boseley, 2003; CEO, 2012). The ILSI now has branches in both China and India, where Big Food companies, including Coca-Cola, are well represented on the Board of Trustees and on Scientific Advisory Committees (ILSI, 2013a, 2013b). In 2006, the World Health Organization barred the ILSI from taking part in activities related to setting food standards because of concerns that the WHO would risk 'scientific credibility and may be compromising public health by partnering with the ILSI' (New Internationalist, 2006). However, in China and India, the ILSI retains strong links to governing organizations. In China, the ILSI has been based in the Chinese Government's Center for Disease Control and Prevention (CDC) (ILSI, 2013a). In India, the ILSI lists as its partners a range of government agencies, including the Ministry of Food Processing Industries, the Ministry of Health, and the Ministry of Rural Development (ILSI, 2014).

Lobbying to resist regulation or urge weak regulation

Brownell and Warner (2009) note how Big Food initially attempts to resist regulation, but when local and state actions turn against them, they instead urge weak national or state action. In the United States, trade organizations like the American Beverage Association (ABA) play a key role in representing the interests of food and beverage companies (Brownell & Warner 2009). In India, Coca-Cola and PepsiCo have put aside their rivalry to form the Indian Beverage Association (IBA). The ABA has served as the model for the IBA, and has also featured prominently in early IBA conferences and meetings (IBA, 2013). Upon its establishment, the IBA was 'tasked with lobbying government on issues of taxation, industry guidelines and regulations, and defending itself against allegations from health activists and environmental campaigners' (Soft Drinks International, 2010).

India serves as a good example of how taxation can be an effective means through which to reduce soft drink consumption. Recent modeling work using household survey data estimates that increasing the tax on soft drinks in the country by 20% could reduce obesity and overweight levels by 3% and diabetes prevalence by 1.6% between 2014 and 2023 (Basu et al., 2014). However, there is also reason to believe that prior state-level tax increases contributed to a reduction in sales. In 2011, the industry cited tax increases as a major factor in PepsiCo and Coca-Cola's slowing growth rates, which at 17 and 8%, respectively, were 'growing considerably slower than two years back when their growth rate was 20–30%' (Bhushan, 2011). One of the most notable tax hikes was in the state of Delhi, which in 2010 increased VAT on soft drinks from 12.5% to 20% (Telegraph, 2010). Just as it has in the US (Kamerow, 2010), the soft drink industry has lobbied against 'soda taxes' in India. Initially, the industry tried to persuade the state government to roll back the hike (FnB News, 2010; Maiti, 2011). The IBA lobbied key political figures, like Delhi Chief Minister Sheila Dikshit (Bhushan, 2010). Dikshit has been a regular invitee at Coca-Cola-sponsored functions, such as those related to the company's Corporate Social Responsibility (CSR) initiatives (Pillai, 2009), their official sponsorship of the 2010 Commonwealth Games in Delhi (Anon, 2010; Coca-Cola India, 2012), and the Coke Studio TV show (Maddox, 2012).

Thus far, the industry has been largely unsuccessful in lobbying against tax increases, with the 2014 budget proposing an additional 5% hike in the excise duty on aerated drinks with added sugar (Times of India, 2014). Recently, the IBA has lobbied more generally in support of a more streamlined tax structure. For over a decade, the Indian Government has been debating the terms of the introduction of a Goods and Services Tax (GST) – a tax that would replace all current state and central indirect taxes on goods and services. The IBA has argued that the beverage industry be made a 'key stakeholder in the introduction of GST and should be a natural partner in the process of consultation while formulating the plan and roll out of GST' (Coca-Cola, 2013). This argument has been made in a number of public venues, including at an IBA-organized seminar attended by key political figures like Shri Rakesh Kacker, Secretary in the Indian Government's Ministry of Food Processing Industries (Coca-Cola, 2013).

In opposition to tax increases, the industry has made three main arguments. Building on Brownell and Warner's (2009) approach, we can draw comparisons between the arguments made by Big Tobacco and the arguments made by Big Food, but can also identify novel arguments made by the latter.

Tobacco companies and tobacco interest groups often argue that their industry is a major supplier of jobs (Saloojee & Dagli, 2000). Also, in the US, the Sugar Association opposed a WHO report on diet and physical activity, on the grounds that limiting intake of dietary sugar would have a detrimental effect on 'the hard working sugar growers and their families' (Brownell & Warner, 2009). The IBA has argued that the industry is a major supplier of jobs, adding that its growth 'will also benefit millions of farmers across the country' (Coca-Cola, 2013). It argued that the Indian Government should 'reverse this hike as it will retard the progress of an industry which can have a significant positive impact on India's development, particularly in the changed governance scenario in the country' (Coca-Cola, 2014). From a public health perspective, although a tax-driven drop in sales could potentially lead to a reduction in job opportunities, this needs to be weighed against the fact that it would also likely lead to a reduction in the cases of obesity and non-communicable disease (Basu et al., 2014).

The tobacco industry has long urged government to reduce taxes on the grounds that it will reduce contraband, counterfeit, and cross-border trade and thus increase revenue (Joossens & Raw, 1995, 2000). Also, in liberalizing countries, where economic policies are in flux, tobacco companies often use this argument when lobbying in favor of their preferred tax structure (Smith, Savell, & Gilmore, 2013). These arguments are often made not only in regards to illicit processes, such as smuggling and bootlegging, but also to processes, where the consumer can legally avoid tax-driven price hikes, such as cross-border shopping. In India, approximately 400 million people are employed in a large 'unorganized sector', which includes small, private, unincorporated sales entities, whose economic activities are difficult for the government to monitor (Ghosh & Ghosh, 2008). The IBA argued that the hike would force the industry

> to increase the price of its products ... [which] will also fuel the growth of beverage options from the spurious and unorganized sector which ... poses significant risk to public health and will take away tax revenue from the Government. (Coca-Cola, 2014)

Research has shown that the tobacco industry often misleadingly argues that tobacco tax and price rises will increase the illicit tobacco trade (Smith et al., 2013). Similarly, independent research on the full extent to which tax-driven price increases fuels the growth of 'spurious' beverage options is needed before such arguments be accepted.

Beverages, unlike tobacco, can provide essential nutrients for health. In opposition to tax increases, the IBA have also argued that 'in a country where options of safe, convenient and hygienic beverages are rather limited, carbonated soft drinks play a very important role in meeting the hydration needs of people' (Coca-Cola, 2014). Thus they argue that the industry should be given 'due recognition as manufacturers of high quality, healthy and nutritious products as well as life critical products like water' (Coca-Cola, 2013).

Experience from tobacco control shows how increasing the taxation, and thus price, of one product type often leads to 'product substitution', where the consumer switches to a similar product, provided the price of the latter has not also increased (Chaloupka, Yurekli, & Fong, 2012). Thus, from a public health perspective, the Indian tax hikes on sugar-added aerated beverages are beneficial, since they could encourage the consumer to switch to healthier products not covered by the tax, like bottled water.

Conclusion

The findings in this article suggest that the general strategies that food and beverage companies use to influence government and key organizations in HICs like the United States are also being used in MICs like China and India. In this study, Brownell and Warner's (2009) 'corporate playbook' served as a useful and transferrable theoretical framework through which to understand the activities and arguments made by Coca-Cola in China and India. Future research should take other components of the framework – e.g. disputing science and 'creating doubt' – and apply them to other countries and contexts in order to assess their transferability.

The study was informed by an extensive analysis of a wide range of documentary materials. One limitation of this study is that unlike research on Big Tobacco, research on Big Food does not have access to internal industry documents. Therefore, any documentary study must rely largely on a critical analysis of documents made-for-public consumption, which may not reveal the extent of industry activities in the same way as internal documents do. Future research on Big Food in MICs should also look to incorporate interview data as a means of triangulating findings in this study.

The findings of this article are important for two reasons. Firstly, they can be used to inform ongoing debates about how to understand and address Big Food's influence on governments and key organizations in China and India, where they already have a significant presence. Secondly, they help inform upstream debates about how to understand and address Big Food's entry into and growth within other emerging or target middle-income markets.

Using Brownell and Warner's (2009) framework, we see that in China and India, Coca-Cola has lobbied US Government officials to influence trade relations between the countries, made financial contributions to political figures, participated in the 'revolving door' between government and industry, funded professional organizations, and lobbied firstly to roll back taxation and secondly to urge greater industry participation in debates over tax restructuring. The study also provided further comparisons between the tobacco and food and beverage industries (Brownell & Warner, 2009; Dorfman, Cheyne, Friedman, Wadud, & Gottilieb, 2012). It is important to agree with the beverage industry, that tobacco and beverages are very different products, with tobacco being 'harmful in any amount' (ABA, 2012). However, from a public health perspective, we can disagree with them that 'there is simply no comparison between soda and tobacco business practices' (ABA, 2012). These similarities are not unexpected, given the fundamental objective of all such companies is to maximize profit to shareholders, something that Brownell and Warner (2009, p. 284) note is common to both tobacco and food. Certainly, arguments made by the beverage industry in India, in opposition to tax increases, are comparable to arguments made in a number of countries to tobacco tax increases. The case of tobacco tax has shown how industry arguments should not be taken at face value (Joossens & Raw, 1995, Smith et al., 2013) and the same may be said of Big Food's arguments.

This study has also identified some ways in which Big Food's strategies provide challenges that are unique to the political and economic environment in MICs like China and India. For example, in India, ongoing uncertainty over the restructuring of the tax system provides a unique opportunity for all stakeholders, including Big Food and public health agencies, to try and influence government debates on taxation. This issue is complex and warrants more attention. Generally speaking, more complex tax systems are seen to undermine the public health impact of taxes (Chaloupka et al., 2012). However, the existing tax system has enabled a number of states in India to raise the VAT on certain soft drinks, thus attenuating sales growth in those areas. If taxation is the key to reducing obesity levels in MICs like India (Basu et al., 2014), then future tax structures should enable governments to maintain tax levels on sugar-added carbonated beverages. Moreover, as the industry argues for a seat at the table to discuss taxation, we should note Brownell's (2012) argument that 'government, foundations, and other powerful institutions should be working for regulation, not collaboration [with Big Food]'. Additionally, corporate lobbying is becoming increasingly influential in countries like China, where it is still a relatively new practice (The Economist, 2001). In India, multinational companies can take advantage of it being virtually unregulated (Giridharadas, 2006). As 'Western' lobbying becomes more common in MICs, ensuring that it is regulated and is transparent becomes increasingly important (Agarwal, 2010).

These comparisons and considerations aside, any study of the growth of Big Food in countries with transitional economies will benefit from an analysis of the strategies used by multinational companies for market entry. As the case of China has shown, strong political connections to HIC political figures and groups can serve to facilitate and sustain a company's incursion into a new market. However, as the case of India has shown, weak political relations between a company and a country are not necessarily insurmountable. Like many multinationals, Coca-Cola has identified the Middle East and Africa as the 'next wave of long-term growth' and as an 'untapped region with significant potential' (Euromonitor, 2013). Some 'major emerging markets', like Vietnam and Iran (Euromonitor, 2013) are MICs with liberalizing economies. Just as Coca-Cola bought its way into the Indian market two decades ago via their acquisitions of Parle brands, the company has recently spent US$1 billion to acquire 50% equity in Aujan Industries, one of the biggest soft drinks companies in the Middle East (Coca-Cola, 2012a). By the end of 2012, thanks to their investment, Coca-Cola (2012a) had already grown by nearly 10%. Despite poor political relations between the US and Iran, the company is already the market leader in the country (with 21.8% of the market share in 2013) and in the Middle East and Africa overall (with 16.1% of the market share in 2013).

As we continue to address global increases in the burden of non-communicable diseases, continued examination and discussion of Big Food's strategies to increase consumption and influence policy is essential before the obesity problem in MICs gets larger still.

Disclosure statement

The author certifies that he has no affiliations with or involvement in any organization or entity with any financial interest. This study was not funded by any funding bodies or agencies.

Acknowledgements

I would like to thank Dr. Kimberly Dienes for her encouragement and review of this paper, and Professor Marion Nestle for her review and encouragement in the wider project within which this work takes place. No specific funding was received for this study.

References

ABA. (2012). Beverage industry responds to PLoS Medicine opinion piece. Retrieved May 17, 2013, from http://www.ameribev.org/news-media/news-releases-statements/more/279/

Agarwal, V. (2010, December 16). What is the future of Lobbying in India? *Wall Street Journal (India)*. Retrieved March 29, 2013, from http://blogs.wsj.com/indiarealtime/2010/12/16/what-is-the-future-of-lobbying-in-india/

Ani. (2014, March 30). Coca-Cola tops most powerful brands list. *News Nation*. Retrieved May 17, from http://www.newsnation.in/article/36943-coca-cola-tops-most-powerful-brands-list.html

Anon. (2010). *Sheila Dikshit asks Delhiites to join CWG celebrations*. Retrieved May 18, 2012, from http://www.hindustantimes.com/News-Feed/Sport/Sheila-Dikshit-asks-Delhiites-tojoin-CWG-celebrations/Article1-607476.aspx

Balarajan, Y., Selvaraj, S., & Subramanian, S. (2011). Health care and equity in India. *Lancet, 337*, 505–515.

Barnetson, D. (1986, October 2). *Cola war fizzing in India*. United Press International.

Basu, S. (2015). The transitional dynamics of caloric ecosystems: Changes in the food supply around the world. *Critical Public Health, 25*. Published Online 27 June 2014. doi:10.1080/09581596.2014.931568

Basu, S., McKee, M., Galea, G., & Stuckler, D. (2013). Relationship of soft drink consumption to global overweight, obesity, and diabetes: A cross-national analysis of 75 countries. *American Journal of Public Health, 103*, 2071–2077.

Basu, S., Vellakkal, S., Agrawal, S., Stuckler, D., Popkin, B., & Ebrahim, S. (2014). Averting obesity and type 2 diabetes in India through sugar-sweetened beverage taxation: An economic-epidemiologic modeling study. *PLoS Medicine, 11*, e1001582. doi:10.1371/journal.pmed.1001582

Bhushan, R. (2010). Coke, Pepsi join hands for beverage association. *The Economic Times (India)*. Retrieved March 12, 2013, from http://articles.economictimes.indiatimes.com/2010-07-05/news/27581124_1_bottlers-energy-drink-maker-iba

Bhushan, R. (2011). PepsiCo sales growing twice as fast as Coca-Cola. *The Economic Times*. Retrieved May 20, 2013, from http://articles.economictimes.indiatimes.com/2011-08-08/news/29864298_1_coca-cola-india-sprite-soft-drinks-market

Boseley, S. (2003, January 9). What are fizzy drinks doing to our children? *The Guardian*. Retrieved April 15, 2012, from http://www.guardian.co.uk/society/2003/jan/09/medicineand health.publichealth

Briggs, H. (2014). *WHO: Daily sugar intake 'should be halved'*. Retrieved November 15, from http://www.bbc.co.uk/news/health-26449497

Brownell, K. (2012). Thinking forward: The quicksand of appeasing the food industry. *PLoS Medicine, 9*, e1001254.

Brownell, K. D., & Warner, K. E. (2009). The perils of ignoring history: Big tobacco played dirty and millions died. How similar is big food? *Milbank Quarterly, 87*, 259–294.

Businessweek. (2014). *Company overview of Coca-Cola India private limited*. Retrieved September 1, from http://investing.businessweek.com/research/stocks/private/board.asp?privcapId= 22818192

Butterfield F. (1979, January 30). Differences fade as rivals mingle to Honor Teng. *NY Times*, p. A1.

Chacon, V., Letona, P., Villamor, E., & Barnoya, J. (2015). Snack food advertising in stores around public schools in Guatamala. *Critical Public Health, 25*. Published online 9 September 2014. doi:10.1080/09581596.2014.953035

Chaloupka, F., Yurekli, A., & Fong, G. (2012). Tobacco taxes as a tobacco control strategy. *Tobacco Control, 21*, 172–180.

Chicago Tribune. (1977, November 21). Coca-Cola thirsts for bigger world sales. *Chicago Tribune*, p. E12.

China Business Review. (2010a). *Dinner honors fifth anniversary of US-China working group*. Retrieved April 15, 2012, from http://www.chinabusinessreview.com/dinner-honors-fifth-anniversary-of-us-china-working-group/

China Business Review. (2010b). *USCBC welcomes PRC Ambassador Zhang Yesui*. Retrieved April 15, 2012, from http://www.chinabusinessreview.com/dinner-honors-fifth-anniversary-of-us-china-working-group/

China Business Review. (2011). *USCBC hosts luncheon honoring PRC vice president Xi Jinping*. Retrieved April 15, 2012, from http://www.chinabusinessreview.com/uscbc-hosts-luncheon-honoring-prc-vice-president-xi-jinping/

Coca-Cola. (2007). *Political contributions reports, 2007*. Retrieved May 10, 2013, from http://politicalaccountability.net/index.php?ht=a/GetDocumentAction/i/7091

Coca-Cola. (2008). *Political contributions reports, 2008*. Retrieved May 10, 2013, from http://politicalaccountability.net/index.php?ht=a/GetDocumentAction/i/7092

Coca-Cola. (2009). *Political contributions reports, 2009*. Retrieved May 10, 2013, from http://politicalaccountability.net/index.php?ht=a/GetDocumentAction/i/7093

Coca-Cola. (2010). *Political contributions reports, 2010*. Retrieved May 10, 2013, from http://politicalaccountability.net/index.php?ht=a/GetDocumentAction/i/7094

Coca-Cola. (2011) *Political contributions reports, 2011*. Retrieved May 10, 2013, from http://assets.coca-colacompany.com/6f/a2/e4469d1848cdab7456acaac4ad9e/2011%20PAC%20and%20Corporate%20Political%20Contributions%20Report.pdf

Coca-Cola. (2012a). *Annual review*. Retrieved March 20, 2013, from http://www.coca-colacompany.com/annualreview/2012/pdf/form_10K_2012.pdf

Coca-Cola. (2012b). *Company history*. Retrieved April 15, 2012, from http://www.cocacolaindia.com/ourcompany/company_history.html

Coca-Cola. (2013). *Press release: The Indian beverage industry will continue to witness double digit growth*. Retrieved January 10, 2014, from http://www.coca-colaindia.com/presscenter/IBA-Growth.html

Coca-Cola. (2014). *Press release: Indian beverage association reacts to the excise duty hike on aerated drinks in the union budget 2014–2015*. Retrieved August 10, from http://www.coca-colaindia.com/presscenter/IBA-reacts.html

Coca-Cola India. (2012). *Newsletter*, p. 3. Retrieved March 12, from http://www.cocacolaindia.com/CMS/Asset/newsletter_old.pdf

Cohen, J. (1986). The dynamics of the 'Revolving Door' on the FCC. *American Journal of Political Science, 30*, 689–708.

Corporate Europe Observatory. (2012). The International Life Sciences Institute (ILSI), Corporate Lobby Group. Retrieved May 12, 2013, from http://corporateeurope.org/sites/default/files/ilsi-articlefinal.pdf

Crossette, B. (1990, February 26). Pepsi is open for business in India. *NY Times*, p. D4.

Dal Bo, E. (2006). Regulatory capture: A review. *Oxford Review of Economic Policy, 22*, 203–225.

Dorfman, L., Cheyne, A., Friedman, L., Wadud, A., & Gottilieb, M. (2012). Soda and tobacco industry corporate social responsibility campaigns: How do they compare? *PLoS Medicine, 9*, e1001241.

Eichenwald, K. (1985, July 16). Soda, the life of the party. *NY Times*, p. A23.

Euromonitor. (2013). The Coca-Cola company in soft drinks (world). Retrieved March 12, from www.euromonitor.com/

Euromonitor International. (2005). *Diet soft drinks see fat growth.* Retrieved March 18, 2012, from www.euromonitor.com/

Euromonitor International. (2010). *What if the Chinese were to spend and drink like Americans.* Retrieved March 29, 2012, from www.euromonitor.com

Euromonitor International. (2011). Global soft drinks: Corporate strategies. Retrieved February 20, 2012, from http://www.euromonitor.com/global-soft-drinks-corporate-strategies/report

Euromonitor International. (2013). *Dataset: Soft drinks.* Retrieved June 5, from www.portal.euro monitor.com

FnB News. (2010, May 7). Soft drink makers in Dehli Want VAT rollback. *FnBNews.com.* Retrieved March 12, 2012, from http://www.fnbnews.com/article/detnew.asp?articleid= 27504&sectionid=3

Ghosh, C., & Ghosh, A. (2008). *Economics of the public sector.* Delhi: PHI Learning.

Gilmore, A. (2005). *Tobacco and transition: Understanding the impact of transition on tobacco use and control in the former soviet union* (PhD in Public Health Medicine). London School of Hygiene & Tropical Medicine, London. Retrieved from http://repositories.cdlib.org/tc/ reports/SovietUnion/

Giridharadas, A. (2006, May 18). India's new lobbyists use american methods. *NY Times*. Online. Retrieved March 12, 2012, from http://www.nytimes.com/2006/05/18/business/worldbusiness/ 18ihtlobby.1778893.html?_r=2&pagewanted=all

Guardino, S. D., & Daynard, R. A. (2007). Tobacco industry lawyers as disease vectors. *Tobacco Control, 16*, 224–228.

Guba, E. (1981). Criteria for assessing the trustworthiness of naturalistic inquiries. *Educational Communication and Technology: A Journal of Theory, Research, and Development, 29*, 75–91.

Gulati, N., & Ahmed, R. (2012). India has 1.2 billion people but not enough drink coke. *The Wall Street Journal.* Retrieved August 29, from http://online.wsj.com/article/ SB10001424052702304870304577490092413939410.html

Igumbor, E. U., Sanders, D., Puoane, T. R., Tsolekile, L., Schwarz, C., Purdy, C., ... Hawkes, C. (2012). 'Big Food', the consumer food environment, health, and the policy response in South Africa. *PLoS Medicine, 9*, e1001253. doi:10.1371/journal.pmed.1001253

Indian Beverage Association. (2013). IBA Conclave. Retrieved March 20, from http://www.inbe verage.org/conclave.htm

India Today. (2014, May 27). Full list of portfolios of ministers in Modi government. *IndiaToday.* Retrieved May 30, from http://indiatoday.intoday.in/story/pm-narendra-modi-cabinet-rajnath-singh-home-arun-jaitley-finance/1/363805.html%20-%20Scene_1

International Life Science Institute, Focal Point in China. (2013a). Retrieved March 20, from http://www.ilsi.org/FocalPointinChina/Pages/AboutUs.aspx

International Life Sciences Institute, India. (2013b). Committee of scientific advisors. Retrieved March 20, from http://www.ilsi-india.org/PDF/ILSI-India%20Expert%20Committees.pdf

International Life Sciences Institute, India. (2014). ILSI-India partners in activities. Retrieved May 15, from http://www.ilsi.org/India/Documents/ILSI-India-Partners-in-Activities.pdf

Jahiel, R. (2008). Corporation-induced diseases, upstream epidemiologic surveillance, and urban health. *Journal of Urban Health, 85*, 517–531.

Jahiel, R., & Babor, T. (2007). Industrial epidemics, public health advocacy and the alcohol industry: Lessons from other fields. *Addiction, 102*, 335–339.

Janofsky, M. (1993, February 25). Coke expand in China, seeking a giant market. *NY Times*, p. D1.

Jensen, M. (1978, April 9). A market thirst never quenched. *NY Times*, p. F1.

Joossens, L., & Raw, M. (1995). Smuggling and cross border shopping of tobacco in Europe. *British Medical Journal, 310*, 1393–1397.

Joossens, L., & Raw, M. (2000). How can cigarette smuggling be reduced? *British Medical Journal, 321*, 947–950.

Kamerow, D. (2010). The case of the sugar sweetened beverage tax. *British Medical Journal, 341*, c3719.

Kellerhals, M. (2012). Congressional leaders meet with China's Xi Jinping. Retrieved September 16, from http://iipdigital.usembassy.gov/st/english/article/2012/02/20120215163018elrem0.2514612.html#axzz21ein02QE

Kelly, B., King, L., Jamiyan, B., Chimedtseren, N., Bold, B., Medina, V., ... Varghese, C. (2015) Density of outdoor food and beverage advertising around schools in Ulaanbaatar (Mongolia) and Manila (The Philippines) and implications for policy. *Critical Public Health, 25*. Published Online 1 August 2014. doi:10.1080/09581596.2014.940850

Kleiman, S., Ng, S., & Popkin, P. (2012). Drinking to our health: Can beverage companies cut calories while maintaining profits? *Obesity Reviews*, 258–274.

Kleinfield N. (1978, December 20) Coca-Cola to go on sale in China as US and Peking expand ties. *NY Times*, p. A1.

Koten, J. (1980, March 5). Problems bubble up at Coca-Cola as Austin prepares to step down. *Wall Street Journal*, p. 1.

Larsen, R. (2013). Committees and caucuses: The US-China working group. Retrieved May 10, from http://larsen.house.gov/legisaltive-work/committees-and-caucuses

Lee, K., & Collin, J. (2006). 'Key to the Future': British American tobacco and cigarette smuggling in China. *PLoS Medicine, 3*, 1080–1089.

Lilien, G., & Yoon, E. (1990). The timing of competitive market entry: An exploratory study of new industrial products. *Management Science, 36*, 568–585.

Lobstein, T. (2014). *Reducing consumption of sugar-sweetened beverages to reduce the risk of childhood overweight and obesity.* Retrieved November 15, from http://www.who.int/elena/titles/commentary/ssbs_childhood_obesity/en/

Maddox, G. (2012). *The good life: Coke studio went live with a power audience.* Retrieved March 20, 2013, from http://www.dailymail.co.uk/indiahome/indianews/article-2165674/The-Good-Life-Coke-Studio-went-live-power-audience-led.html

Maiti, M. (2011). Coca-Cola feels the heat. *Financial Chronicle*. Retrieved May 20, 2013, from http://www.mydigitalfc.com/news/coca-cola-feels-heat-935

Makkai, T., & Braithwaite, J. (1992). In and out of the revolving door: Making sense of regulatory capture. *Journal of Public Policy, 12*, 61–78.

McNulty T. (1979, February 1). Teng's tour: A tiny slice of America: Chopstick-proof meals in a three-city visit. *Chicago Tribune*, p. 1.

Mok, V., Dai, X., & Yeung, G. (2002). An Internalization approach to joint ventures: Coca-Cola in China. *Asia Pacific Business Review, 9*, 39–58.

Monteiro, C. A., & Cannon, G. (2012). The impact of transnational 'Big Food' companies on the south: A view from Brazil. *PLoS Medicine, 9*, e1001252. doi:10.1371/journal.pmed.1001252

Nestle, M. (2002). *Food politics: How the food industry influences nutrition and health.* Berkeley, CA: University of California Press.

Nestlé (Company). (2011). *Annual report.* Retrieved May 20, 2012, from http://www.nestle.com/Common/NestleDocuments/Documents/Library/Documents/Annual_Reports/2011-Annual-Report-EN.pdf

New Internationalist. (2006). Corporate No-No. Issue 388. Retrieved May 20, 2013, from http://newint.org/columns/currents/2006/04/01/corporate/

Nolan, P. (1996). Large firms and industrial reform in former planned economies: The case of China. *Cambridge Journal of Economics, 20*, 1–29.

NY Times. (1977, September 5). India stands firm against Coca-Cola. *NY Times*, p. 22.

NY Times. (1990, March 22). Coca-Cola rebuffed by India. *NY Times*, p. D20.

Orleans, C., & Slade, J. (1993). *Nicotine addiction: Principles and management.* New York, NY: Oxford University Press.

Pendergrast, M. (2000). *For god, country & Coca-Cola: The definitive history of the great American soft drink and the company that makes it.* New York, NY: Basic Books.

PepsiCo. (2011). *Annual report.* Retrieved May 20, 2012, from http://www.pepsico.com/annual11/downloads/PEP_AR11_2011_Annual_Report.pdf

Pillai, S. (2009, July 16). For a better tomorrow. *The Hindu.* Retrieved May 17, 2012, from http://www.hindu.com/mp/2009/07/16/stories/2009071651610300.htm

Pingali, P. (2007). Westernization of Asian diets and the transformation of food systems: Implications for research and policy. *Food Policy, 32,* 385–393.

Popkin, B. (2012). Global nutrition transition and the pandemic of obesity in developing countries. *Nutrition Reviews, 70,* 3–21.

Rangan, K. (1977, August 9). *New York Times,* p. 45.

Ritchie, J., & Spencer, L. (2002). Qualitative data analysis in applied policy research. In A. M. Huberman & M. B. Miles (Eds.), *The qualitative researcher's companion* (pp. 305–331). London: Sage.

Sahu, P., & Kala, A. (2014, May 27). Meet the man who will try to fix India's economy. *The Wall Street Journal.* Retrieved May 28, from http://blogs.wsj.com/indiarealtime/2014/05/27/meet-the-man-who-will-try-to-fix-indias-economy/

Saloojee, Y., & Dagli, E. (2000). Tobacco industry tactics for resisting public policy on health. *Bulletin of the World Health Organization, 78,* 902–910.

Shenton, A. (2004). Strategies for ensuring trustworthiness in qualitative research projects. *Education for Information, 22,* 63–75.

Shirane, R., Smith, K., Ross, H., Silver, K. E., Williams, S., & Gilmore, A. (2012). Tobacco industry manipulation of tobacco excise and tobacco advertising policies in the Czech Republic: An analysis of tobacco industry documents. *PLoS Medicine, 9,* e100124868.

Smith, K., Fooks, G., Collin, J., Weishaar, H., & Gilmore, A. (2010). Is the increasing policy use of Impact assessment in Europe likely to undermine efforts to achieve healthy public policy? *Journal of Epidemiology and Community Health, 64,* 478–487.

Smith, K., Savell, E., & Gilmore, A. (2013). What is known about tobacco industry efforts to influence tobacco tax? A systematic review of empirical studies. *Tobacco Control, 22,* 144–153.

Soft Drinks International. (2010, August). *India: Beverage association is formed. Soft drinks international,* p. 16. Wimborne: ASAP Publishing.

Sterba, J. (1981, April 16). Coke brings 'tasty happiness' to China. *NY Times,* p. A1.

Stuckler, D., McKee, M., Ebrahim, S., & Basu, S. (2012). Manufacturing epidemics: The role of global producers in increased consumption of unhealthy commodities including processed foods, alcohol, and tobacco. *PLoS Medicine, 9,* e1001235.

Stuckler, D., & Nestle, M. (2012). Big food, food systems, and global health. *PLoS Medicine, 9,* e1001242. doi:10.1371/journal.pmed.1001242

Taylor, F., Satija, A., Khurana, S., Singh, G., & Ebrahim, S. (2010). Pepsi and Coca Cola in Delhi, India: Availability, price and sales. *Public Health Nutrition, 14,* 653–660.

Telegraph. (2010, July 7). Beverage brethren uncork spirit of unity. *The Telegraph (India).* Retrieved May 19, 2012, from http://www.telegraphindia.com/1100707/jsp/business/story_12654979.jsp

The Economist. (2001, February 15). The gentle art of lobbying in China. Retrieved May 15, 2013, from http://www.economist.com/node/505497

Times of India. (2014, July 10). Highlights of union budget 2014. *Times of India.* Retrieved July 11, from http://timesofindia.indiatimes.com/budget-2014/union-budget-2014/Highlights-of-Union-Budget-2014/articleshow/38115864.cms

US-China Business Council. (2010, June 2). The US-China business council elects the coca-cola company chairman and CEO Muhtar Kent as Chair; welcomes new board members, officers.

Press release. Retrieved March 15, 2012, from https://www.uschina.org/public/documents/2010/06/uscbc-elections.html

US-India Business Council. (2012a). *The way forward: Business advocacy Agenda*. Retrieved August 19, from http://www.usibc.com/sites/default/files/advocacy/files/17148_TheWayForward_NoCrop.pdf

US-China Business Council. (2012b). *2012 Meetings and events*. Retrieved March 15, from https://www.uschina.org/info/programs/recentpastevents.html

Washington Post. (1979, January 24). A half million cokes rolling into China. *The Washington Post*, p. D7.

Weisert, D. (2001, July–August). Coca-Cola in China: Quenching the thirst of a billion. *China Business Review*. Retrieved August 15, 2012, from https://www.chinabusinessreview.com/public/0107/weisert.html

Weisman, S. (1988, March 21). Pepsi sets off a Cola war in India. *NY Times*, p. D12.

World Health Organization. (2014). *WHO opens public consultation on draft sugars guideline*. Retrieved November 15, from http://www.who.int/mediacentre/news/notes/2014/consultation-sugar-guideline/en/

Comparison of food industry policies and commitments on marketing to children and product (re)formulation in Australia, New Zealand and Fiji

Gary Sacks[a], Melissa Mialon[a], Stefanie Vandevijvere[b], Helen Trevena[c],
Wendy Snowdon[a,d], Michelle Crino[c] and Boyd Swinburn[a,b]

[a]WHO Collaborating Centre for Obesity Prevention, Deakin University, Victoria, Australia;
[b]School of Population Health, University of Auckland, Auckland, New Zealand; [c]The George
Institute for Global Health, University of Sydney, Sydney, Australia; [d]Pacific Research Centre for
the Prevention of Obesity and Non-communicable Diseases (C-POND), Suva, Fiji

Unhealthy food environments are known to be major drivers of diet-related
non-communicable diseases globally, and there is an imperative for major
food companies to be publicly accountable for their actions to improve the
healthiness of food environments. This paper examines the prevalence of publicly available policies and commitments of major packaged food and soft
drink manufacturers, and fast-food restaurants in Australia, New Zealand and
Fiji with respect to reducing food marketing to children and product (re)for-
mulation. In each country, the most prominent companies in each sector were
selected. Company policies, commitments and relevant industry initiatives
were gleaned from company and industry association websites. In Australia
and New Zealand, there are a higher proportion of companies with publicly
available marketing and formulation policies than in Fiji. However, even in
Australia, a large proportion of the most prominent food companies do not
have publicly available policies. Where they exist, policies on food marketing
to children generally focus on those aged less than 12, do not apply to all
types of media, marketing channels and techniques, and do not provide transparency with respect to the products to which the policies apply. Product formulation policies, where they exist, focus mostly on salt reduction and
changes to the make-up of overall product portfolios, and do not generally
address saturated fat, added sugar and energy reduction. In the absence of
strong policies and corresponding actions by the private sector, it is likely that
government action (e.g. through co-regulation or legislation) will be needed to
drive improved company performance.

Background

Unhealthy food environments are known to be major drivers of obesity and diet-related
non-communicable diseases (NCDs) globally (World Health Organization, 2011). Private sector organisations, including all industry stakeholders involved in producing,
packaging, distributing and marketing food products and beverages (collectively referred
to as 'the food industry'), are critical in shaping the food environments of individuals

and populations (Sacks et al., 2013; World Health Organization, 2004). While the food industry has been criticised for its part in making food environments less healthy over recent decades (Brownell & Horgen, 2004; Brownell & Warner, 2009; Moodie et al., 2013; Nestle, 2002; The PLoS Medicine Editors, 2012), it is also widely acknowledged that the food industry has the collective power to be a major contributor to making food environments healthier (Gortmaker et al., 2011; United Nations, 2011; World Health Organization, 2004).

Two of the main areas in which the food industry can play an active role in improving the healthiness of food environments are: (1) reducing marketing of unhealthy food products and non-alcoholic beverages to children (hereafter, food marketing to children), and (2) formulation and reformulation of products to improve their nutrition composition (e.g. reduce salt, saturated fat, *trans* fat, added sugar, energy) (hereafter, product formulation). Leading international and national health organisations, including the World Health Organization (WHO), the World Cancer Research Fund and the United States Institute of Medicine (IOM), identify recommendations for the private sector with respect to food marketing to children and product formulation (see Table 1). In addition, the WHO highlights the importance of independent and transparent monitoring of policies and commitments made by the private sector at national and global levels (World Health Organization, 2010). The Access to Nutrition Index (ATNI), a monitoring initiative that evaluates food and beverage manufacturers on their nutrition-related commitments, disclosure practices and performance related to obesity and undernutrition, includes specific benchmarks for companies in relation to food marketing to children and product formulation, amongst other categories (Access to Nutrition Index, 2013). With respect to food marketing to children, ATNI's key recommendations are for each company to: establish and implement a single policy on marketing to children that is comprehensive in its scope and is applied to all media channels and markets in which they operate; prioritise healthier products in their marketing investments, and provide quantitative substantiation of such efforts; and commission independent, external audits of compliance with their own policies on a regular basis, and disclose these results. With respect to product formulation, ATNI's key recommendations are for each company to set targets to improve the formulation of products across their entire portfolio, and disclose targets and performance in a consistent way that is easy to understand.

In many countries, the sectors of the food industry that are most prominent and influential are packaged food manufacturers (including large retailers that supply non-branded, or 'private-brand', products), soft drink manufacturers and fast food restaurants. Within these sectors, the largest companies typically include a mix of multinational and national companies. Globally, governments have generally relied on industry self-regulation in order to reduce food marketing to children (International Association for the Study of Obesity [IASO], 2010) and improve product formulation (Neal et al., 2013). Some companies are taking concerted actions to improve food environments (Access to Nutrition Index, 2013), typically in response to pressure from consumer groups, and government or non-government organisations (NGOs) in some high-income countries (Brinsden et al., 2013). However, there is concern that current industry self-regulatory approaches are insufficient to address the problem (Elliott et al., 2014; Lumley, Martin, & Antonopoulos, 2012). Furthermore, there is concern that, even when multinational companies make improvements in high-income countries, they do not apply those actions across all of the countries in which they operate, particularly in low- and middle-income countries where there is often less pressure from civil society groups and weaker accountability mechanisms (Monteiro, Gomes, & Cannon, 2010).

Table 1. Globally recommended actions (from selected authoritative reports) for the private sector with respect to food marketing and product reformulation.

Report	Recommended actions for the private sector with respect to food marketing	Recommended actions for the private sector with respect to product reformulation
World Health Organization (WHO) Global Strategy for Diet and Physical Activity (DPAS) (World Health Organization, 2004)	• Practise responsible marketing that supports DPAS, particularly with regard to the promotion and marketing of foods high in saturated fats, trans-fatty acids, free sugars or salt, especially to children • Promote healthy diets and physical activity in accordance with national guidelines, international standards and the overall aims of DPAS	• Continue to develop and provide affordable, healthy and nutritious choices to consumers • Limit the levels of saturated fats, trans-fatty acids, free sugars and salt in existing products, and consider introducing new products with better nutritional value • Provide information on food composition to national authorities
WHO set of recommendations on the marketing of foods and non-alcoholic beverages to children (World Health Organization, 2010)	• Private sector stakeholders should be encouraged to follow marketing practices that are consistent with the WHO recommendations and to practise them globally in order to ensure equal consideration to children everywhere and avoid undermining efforts to restrict marketing in countries that receive food marketing from beyond their borders	• Not applicable
WHO Global Action Plan for the Prevention and Control of Non-communicable diseases 2013–2020 (World Health Organization, 2013)	• Take measures to implement the WHO set of recommendations to reduce the impact of the marketing of unhealthy foods and non-alcoholic beverages to children, while taking into account existing national legislation and policies	• Consider producing and promoting more food products consistent with a healthy diet, including by reformulating products to provide healthier options that are affordable and accessible and that follow relevant nutrition facts and labelling standards, including information on sugars, salt and fats, and where appropriate, trans-fat content

(Continued)

Table 1. (*Continued*).

Report	Recommended actions for the private sector with respect to food marketing	Recommended actions for the private sector with respect to product reformulation
		• Work towards reducing the use of salt in the food industry in order to lower sodium consumption
Institute of Medicine Food Marketing to Children and Youth: Threat or Opportunity (Institute of Medicine, 2006)	• Advertise and market products that are substantially lower in total energy, fats, salt and added sugars, and have a higher positive nutrient content • Work with government, health professionals and consumer groups to revise, expand, enforce and evaluate self-regulatory guidelines to include all forms of marketing and communications (e.g. social media, games as well as traditional print and television)	• Shift the product portfolio to foods that are lower in total energy, fats, salts and added sugars, and have a higher positive nutrient content
World Cancer Research Fund (WCRF) Policy and Action for Cancer Prevention (World Cancer Research Fund/ American Institute for Cancer Research, 2009)	• Collaborate in order to stop advertising, promotion and easy availability of sugary drinks and unhealthy foods to children • Ensure accuracy, uniformity and availability of product information in all advertising and promotion and on food labels	• Make public health an explicit priority in all stages of food systems including product research, development, formulation and reformulation, and promotion

This paper examines the publicly available policies and commitments of the major packaged food manufacturers, soft drink manufacturers and fast-food restaurants in three countries in the Pacific region (Australia, New Zealand and Fiji) with respect to food marketing to children and product formulation. The paper aims to compare the prevalence of publicly available policies and commitments, including broad comparisons across sectors and countries, with reference to globally recommended actions for the private sector in each domain. This includes a comparison of policies in high-income countries (Australia and New Zealand) to those in a middle-income country (Fiji) in the same region. Detailed assessment of individual company policies, and an examination of the way in which company policies are translated into action (e.g. actual marketing to children and product nutrition composition changes) are beyond the scope of this paper.

Methods

Selection of companies

In each country, the selection of companies for inclusion in the analysis was based on the approach recommended by INFORMAS (International Network for Food and Obesity/NCDs Research, Monitoring and Action Support) for determining 'organisations of interest' for monitoring private sector policies and practices related to food environments (Sacks et al., 2013). INFORMAS recommends that monitoring activities are prioritised to focus on the sectors within the food industry that pose the greatest threat and/or have the greatest opportunity to improve public health nutrition, and the most prominent food companies in each sector should be selected by taking into account market share, products and services provided, and levels of influence (Sacks et al., 2013).

For Australia and New Zealand, the Euromonitor International Passport database (Euromonitor International, 2013) was used to determine company market share (by revenue) in different sectors of the food industry for 2012. All packaged food companies that had >1% market share were selected. Within this sector, the Euromonitor database separately identified market share information related to 'private-label' products (i.e. as used by supermarkets). Where the market share related to private-label products was >1%, the largest grocery store-based retailers (with >20% market share) were also selected for analysis. All soft drinks manufacturers that had >5% market share, and all fast food restaurants that had >3% market share were also selected. The market share percentages in each sector were selected to ensure that at least 50% of the market in each sector was included.

For Fiji, due to the absence of Euromonitor (or equivalent) data related to market share, the most prominent packaged food companies were selected based on the most prominent products in the most recent (2002) National Nutrition Survey (Ministry of Health, 2007) and in-store surveys (Snowdon et al., 2013). The five largest soft drink manufacturers, covering 85% of the Fijian market (according to these manufacturers (Fiji Beverages Group, 2014)), and all fast-food restaurants with >1 outlet in Fiji were also selected.

Data collection

An internet search was conducted to locate the website for each of the selected companies in each country. Where possible, the country-specific website for the company was used (e.g. *company.com.au* or *company.co.nz*) to locate country-specific information. In addition, or where no country-specific company website was found, the global website for the company (e.g. *company.com*) was used, where available. Where applicable, searches were also conducted for the websites of major subsidiary companies to the selected companies. In addition, searches were conducted for the websites of the most prominent brands of the selected companies, and other websites directly affiliated with the selected companies. Only webpages related to the food and non-alcoholic beverage divisions of each company were investigated.

Every section of each of the selected company websites were thoroughly searched for information on the company's policy with respect to: (1) food marketing to children and (2) product formulation, including references to efforts to change salt, added sugar, fat (including saturated fat and/or *trans* fat), kilojoule content, and the healthiness of the product portfolio overall. In this context, company 'policy' was defined as 'a stated position, objective, or plan to manage' the issue (The Consumer Goods Forum, 2013). Where applicable, information on company commitments or pledges in each of the two domains was also noted. Where available online, annual financial reports and corporate social responsibility reports were also examined for relevant information.

In each country and at the global-level, industry initiatives with respect to food marketing to children and product formulation were examined. These were identified based on information obtained from individual company websites, websites of NGOs (e.g. the Heart Foundation), industry associations, and the Rudd Center database of food company pledges (Yale Rudd Center for Food Policy and Obesity, 2014). All websites were searched by two of the authors independently, and any discrepancies in results were reviewed by a third author. All website data were valid as of 28 February 2014.

Data analysis

For each of the selected companies in each country, the presence or absence of a policy in each domain (food marketing to children and product formulation) was noted, including whether the policy was detailed on the company's website at the country level or global level (if applicable). A policy was deemed to be present in each domain if a specific reference to a company policy was found or a specific commitment was detailed. If the company was a signatory to a country-level or global-level industry initiative, this was also noted, along with details of the relevant initiative. Where relevant, a company's country-level policies and commitments were compared to their global-level policies and commitments.

With respect to food marketing to children, the content of each company's policy was broadly assessed in relation to the age of the audience, the types of products, the types of media, and the marketing channels and techniques to which the policy applies. With respect to product formulation, the content of each company's policy was broadly assessed in relation to whether the policy addressed salt, fat (including saturated fat and/or *trans* fat), added sugar and / or energy (kJ) reductions, as well as whether reference was made to improving the nutrition composition of the company's overall product portfolio (e.g. through introducing new, healthier products). All results are reported as percentages by sector, within each country. All coding of results was conducted by two of the authors independently, and any discrepancies in coding were reviewed by a third author.

Results

The companies selected for analysis in each country, including their respective market shares in each sector (Australia and New Zealand only), are listed in Table 2. For Australia, 20 packaged food manufacturers were selected, accounting for 63% of market share (by revenue). In addition, the two largest Australian grocery store-based retailers (Woolworths Ltd and Wesfarmers Ltd, not shown in Table 2) were also included, as 'private-label' brands account for an additional 13% of market share in the packaged food manufacturers sector. Five soft drink manufacturers (accounting for 71% of market share) and five fast-food restaurants (accounting for 54% of market share) were included. For New Zealand, 16 packaged food manufacturers were selected, accounting for 73% of market share (by revenue). In addition, the two largest New Zealand

Table 2. Companies selected for analysis in Australia, New Zealand and Fiji.

Sector[1]	Australia Company name (market share in 2012, based on Euromonitor data (Euromonitor International, 2013))	New Zealand Company name (market share in 2012, based on Euromonitor data (Euromonitor International, 2013))	Fiji Company name
Packaged food manufacturers	Kirin Holdings Co Ltd (6.1%)	**Fonterra Co-operative Group** (13.9%)	**Australasian Conference Association Ltd**
	Nestlé S.A. (5.7%)	**Goodman Fielder Ltd** (13.0%)	BBC
	Mondelez International Inc (4.8%)	**H J Heinz Co** (5.8%)	C.J. Patel
	Unilever Group (3.5%)	Mondelez International Inc (4.6%)	FMF Foods Ltd
	Campbell Soup Co (3.4%)	Griffins Foods Ltd (3.1%)	**Fonterra Co-operative Group**
	Mars Inc (3.2%)	**Unilever Group** (3.1%)	Foods Pacific Ltd
	Goodman Fielder Ltd (2.8%)	**Nestlé S.A.** (2.9%)	Foods Processors Ltd
	Groupe Lactalis (2.7%)	Mars Inc (2.3%)	**Goodman Fielder Ltd**
	J R Simplot Co (2.3%)	PepsiCo Inc (2.2%)	**H J Heinz Co**
	Associated British Foods Plc (2.1%)	Campbell Soup Co (2.2%)	Lees Trading Co Ltd
	PepsiCo Inc (2.0%)	Associated British Foods Plc (2.1%)	**Nestlé S.A.**
	H J Heinz Co (1.7%)	**Australasian Conference Association Ltd** (1.8%)	PAFCO
	Kellogg Co (1.6%)	Sealord Group Ltd (1.4%)	Tahi Pacific
	Fonterra Co-operative Group (1.6%)	Danone, Groupe (1.3%)	**Unilever Group**
	McCain Foods Ltd (1.3%)	Kellogg Co (1.2%)	Wallson Foods Ltd
	Australasian Conference Association Ltd (1.1%)	General Mills Inc (1.1%)	
	Kraft Foods Group, Inc (1.0%)		
	Murray Goulburn Co-operative Co Ltd (1.0%)		
	Regal Cream Products Pty Ltd (1.0%)		
	General Mills Inc (1.0%)		
Soft drink manufacturers	The Coca-Cola Co (33.8%)	The Coca-Cola Co (49.1%)	Frezco Beverages Ltd
	Asahi Group Holdings Ltd (13.1%)	Suntory Holdings Ltd (24.5%)	Motibhai Group of Companies
	Kirin Holdings Co Ltd (9.6%)	PepsiCo Inc (4.6%)	Pinto Beverages Ltd
	PepsiCo Inc (8.5%)		Tappoo Group of Companies
	H J Heinz Co (5.6%)		CocaCola Amatil Fiji

(*Continued*)

Table 2. (*Continued*).

Sector[1]	Australia Company name (market share in 2012, based on Euromonitor data (Euromonitor International, 2013))	New Zealand Company name (market share in 2012, based on Euromonitor data (Euromonitor International, 2013))	Fiji Company name
Fast food restaurants	**McDonald's Corp** (25.8%)	**McDonald's Corp** (18.0%)	Chicken Express
	Yum! Brands Inc (11.1%)	Yum! Brands Inc (12.9%)	**McDonald's Corp**
	Doctor's Associates Inc (7.4%)	Doctor's Associates Inc (10.7%)	MH Secret Recipe
	Burger King Worldwide Inc (5.4%)	Burger King Worldwide Inc (8.7%)	Nando's
	Quick Service Restaurant Holdings Pty Ltd (4.5%)	Noodle Canteen Ltd (3.0%)	Wishbone / Pizza King

[1]Companies that were included in all three countries are highlighted in bold.

grocery store-based retailers (Woolworths Ltd and Foodstuffs NZ Ltd, not shown in Table 2) were also included, as 'private-label' brands account for an additional 11% of market share in the packaged food manufacturers sector. Three soft drink manufacturers (accounting for 78% of market share) and five fast-food restaurants (accounting for 53% of market share) were included. For Fiji, 15 packaged food manufacturers, five soft drink manufacturers and five fast-food restaurants were included. Grocery store-based retailers were not included, as 'private-label' brands do not make up a substantial proportion of products purchased in Fiji. In all countries, the selected companies include a mix of national and multinational companies, with a diversity of ownership structures and size. In total, seven companies (highlighted in bold in Table 2) were included in the selection of companies in all three countries.

Food marketing to children

An overview of the policies of the selected companies relating to food marketing to children, for each country and sector, is presented in Table 3. In Australia, 55% of the selected packaged food manufacturers had a policy related to food marketing to children available on the company website. This is a similar level to New Zealand (67%), but substantially higher than Fiji (27%). Similarly, a high percentage of the selected Australian and New Zealand soft drink manufacturers (100 and 67%, respectively) had policies on their websites, whereas none of the selected Fijian soft drink manufacturers had policies on their websites (although all of them were signatories to a national food marketing initiative, see below). Only 20% of the selected Fijian and New Zealand fast food restaurants had online food marketing policies, compared to 60% for Australia.

In Australia, many of the selected companies were signatories to national industry initiatives related to food marketing to children. These include the Australian Food and Grocery Council (AFGC)'s Responsible Children Marketing Initiative (RCMI) (Australian Food and Grocery Council, 2014b) (16 of the 18 signatories to the RCMI are included in the selected companies for Australia), the AFGC's Quick Service Restaurant Initiative for Responsible Advertising and Marketing to Children (QSR) (Australian Food and Grocery

Table 3. Overview of policies and commitments related to food marketing to children for selected companies in Australia, New Zealand and Fiji.

	% of selected companies			Conditions to which policy applies (% of selected companies)[1]						
	Policy on company website (%)	Signatories to national industry-initiatives (%)	Signatories to global industry-initiatives (%)	Audience age (%)		Products[2]		Types of media[3]		Marketing channels and techniques[4]
Australia										
Packaged food manufacturers (including two major retailers)	55	64	36	Age <6 only	0%	Products not specified	22%	All types of media	59%	Interactive games 68%
				Age <12 only	73%	Nutrient profiling criteria (in-house)	41%	All with some exceptions	5%	Schools 68%
				Age not specified	0%	Nutrient profiling criteria (independent)	9%	Not specified	9%	Personalities or characters 23%
				No policy	27%	No policy	27%	No policy	27%	
Soft drink manufacturers	100	100	100	Age <6 only	0%	Products not specified	0%	All types of media	100%	Interactive games 40%
				Age <12 only	100%	Nutrient profiling criteria (in-house)	60%	All with some exceptions	0%	Schools 100%
				Age not specified	0%	Nutrient profiling criteria (independent)	40%	Not specified	0%	Personalities or characters 100%
				No policy	0%	No policy	0%	No policy	0%	

(Continued)

Table 3. (Continued).

	% of selected companies			Conditions to which policy applies (% of selected companies)[1]			
	Policy on company website (%)	Signatories to national industry-initiatives (%)	Signatories to global industry-initiatives (%)	Audience age (%)	Products[2]	Types of media[3]	Marketing channels and techniques[4]
Fast food restaurants	60	100	20	Age <6 only 0% Age <14 only[5] 100% Age not specified 0% No policy 0%	Products not specified 40% Nutrient profiling criteria (in-house) 60% Nutrient profiling criteria (independent) 0% No policy 0%	All types of media 80% All with some exceptions 0% Not specified 20% No policy 0%	Interactive games 100% Schools 100% Personalities or characters 20%
New Zealand Packaged food manufacturers (including two major retailers)	67	6	39	Age <6 only 0% Age <12 only 56% Age not specified 17% No policy 27%	Products not specified 17% Nutrient profiling criteria (in-house) 56% Nutrient profiling criteria (independent) 0% No policy 27%	All types of media 34% All with some exceptions 12% Not specified 28% No policy 27%	Interactive games 0% Schools 50% Personalities or characters 22%

			Age <6 only	Age <12 only	Age not specified	No policy	Products not specified	Nutrient profiling criteria (in-house)	Nutrient profiling criteria (independent)	No policy	All types of media	All with some exceptions	Not specified	No policy	Interactive games	Schools	Personalities or characters
Soft drink manufacturers	67	0	0%	67%	0%	33%	0%	67%	0%	33%	0%	67%	0%	33%	0%	67%	67%
Fast food restaurants	20	0	0%	0%	20%	80%	20%	0%	0%	80%	20%	0%	0%	80%	0%	20%	20%
Fiji																	
Packaged food manufacturers	27	0	0%	20%	7%	73%	13%	13%	0%	73%	13%	13%	0%	73%	0%	20%	20%

(Continued)

Table 3. (Continued).

	% of selected companies			Conditions to which policy applies (% of selected companies)[1]			
	Policy on company website (%)	Signatories to national industry-initiatives (%)	Signatories to global industry-initiatives (%)	Audience age (%)	Products[2]	Types of media[3]	Marketing channels and techniques[4]
Soft drink manufacturers	0	100	20	Age <6 only 0% Age <12 only 100% Age not specified 0% No policy 0%	Products not specified 80% Nutrient profiling criteria (in-house) 20% Nutrient profiling criteria (independent) 0% No policy 0%	All types of media 100% All with some exceptions 0% Not specified 0% No policy 0%	Interactive games 0% Schools 20% Personalities or characters 20%
Fast food restaurants	20	0	20	Age <6 only 0% Age <12 only 20% Age not specified 0% No policy 80%	Products not specified 0% Nutrient profiling criteria (in-house) 20% Nutrient profiling criteria (independent) 0% No policy 80%	All types of media 20% All with some exceptions 0% Not specified 0% No policy 80%	Interactive games 0% Schools 20% Personalities or characters 20%

[1]For each company, the relevant policy includes an amalgamation of policies or commitments specified by the company at the country level, the global level and any industry initiative to which the company is a signatory. In instances where there was a lack of clarity about which of these aspects to infer as the policy of the company, preference was given to data at the country level, with more detailed data deemed to override more general data.

2 'Nutrient profiling criteria (in-house)' refers to criteria developed by the company itself for determining the products to which aspects of their policy apply. 'Nutrient profiling criteria (independent)' refers to criteria developed independently for determining the products to which aspects of their policy apply, including reference to national standards or dietary guidelines.

3 'All types of media' refers to broadcast (television and radio), print and digital media (including internet and phone messaging). 'All with some exceptions' refers to policies that apply to most types of media, but with some exceptions specified.

4 The most common marketing channels and techniques specifically identified as part of company policies were interactive games, schools and personalities or characters. Note that percentages shown in this column do not add up to 100%, as an individual company policy may identify none or many marketing channels and techniques.

5 All of the selected fast food companies in Australia specified that their policies apply to those aged less than 14.

Council, 2014a) (all five of the signatories to the QSR are included in the selected companies for Australia), and the commitments of the Australian Beverages Council (Australian Beverages Council, 2014). In addition, food marketing was self-regulated, including through the Australian Association of National Advertisers' (AANA's) voluntary guidelines for advertising directed at children (AANA, 2013) and various other voluntary advertising industry codes of practice, e.g. the Code of Practice on Nutrient Claims (Australian Food and Grocery Council, 1995). In New Zealand and Fiji, national industry initiatives related to food marketing were less prominent. In New Zealand, food marketing was self-regulated by the Advertising Standards Authority (ASA) through the Children's Code For Advertising Food 2010 (Advertising Standards Authority, 2010), but there are no industry-wide policies or commitments similar to the Australian RCMI or QSR. In Fiji, the newly formed Fiji Beverage Group, including all five of the selected soft drink manufacturers, had entered into a Memorandum of Understanding which includes a commitment to restrict food marketing to children (Fiji Beverages Group, 2014). In all three countries, many of the selected companies were signatories to global industry initiatives such as the International Food and Beverage Alliance (IFBA) Global Policy on Advertising and Marketing Communications to Children (International Food and Beverage Alliance, 2011) and the International Council of Beverages Associations Guidelines on Marketing to Children (International Council of Beverages Associations, 2012). For many of the selected companies, this resulted in a multilayered policy, including policies specified at the global and country levels in addition to commitments through national and global industry initiatives. For example, for Nestle in Australia, their food marketing policy was specified at the global level (Nestle, 2014b), the country level (Nestle, 2014a) and through their affiliations with RCMI and IFBA. For some multinational companies (e.g. The CocaCola Co), a policy was specified at the global level, but no mention of that policy was made on the country-level company website. Similarly, there are many cases in which companies were signatories to industry initiatives, but did not include that information on their country-level company websites.

Across all three countries, where packaged food manufacturers specified an age to which marketing restrictions apply, the majority refer to children under 12 years of age. Across all three countries and all sectors, only a small minority of companies used independent nutrient-profiling criteria to specify which of their products were eligible to be marketed to children, and almost all of the companies that used in-house nutrient-profiling criteria did not disclose the details of their in-house criteria. There is great variety in the extent to which companies specified the types of media and the marketing channels and techniques to which their policies applied. However, in general, the policies of the Australian companies were more specific than those for New Zealand and Fiji. Refer to Table 3 for further details.

For the most part, the seven companies that were included in the selection for all three countries each maintained consistent policies across Australia, New Zealand and Fiji. In most cases, their policies were specified at the global level. Small differences in company policy across the three countries reflected the fact that these companies were taking part in national-level industry initiatives.

Product formulation

An overview of the policies of the selected companies relating to product formulation, for each country and sector, are presented in Table 4. Across the three countries, the percentage of the selected companies with online product formulation policies followed

Table 4. Overview of policies and commitments related to product formulation for selected companies in Australia, New Zealand and Fiji.

	% of selected companies			Content area incorporated in the policy/commitment (% of selected companies)[1]				
	Policy on company website (%)	Signatories to national industry-initiatives (%)	Signatories to global industry-initiatives (%)	Salt reduction (%)	Saturated and /or *trans* fat reduction (%)	Added sugar reduction (%)	Energy (kJ) reduction (%)	Improvements in the overall product portfolio (%)
Australia								
Packaged food manufacturers (including two major retailers)	59	23	36	55	36	14	23	50
Soft drink manufacturers	60	100	40	0	20	0	20	100
Fast food restaurants	80	0	20	60	40	20	0	60
New Zealand								
Packaged food manufacturers (including two major retailers)	72	22	44	67	44	17	6	44
Soft drink manufacturers	33	0	67	33	33	0	0	67
Fast food restaurants	20	0	20	40	20	0	0	20
Fiji								
Packaged food manufacturers	27	0	13	20	13	13	0	27
Soft drink manufacturers	0	100	20	20	20	0	0	100
Fast food restaurants	20	0	20	20	20	0	0	20

[1]For each company, the relevant policy includes an amalgamation of policies or commitments specified by the company at the country level, the global level and any industry initiative to which the company is a signatory. In instances where there was a lack of clarity about which of these aspects to infer as the policy of the company, preference was given to data at the country level, with more detailed data deemed to override more general data.

a similar pattern to the food marketing policies discussed in the section above. For packaged food manufacturers, 59% of the selected Australian companies had policies on their company websites, compared to 72% in New Zealand and 27% in Fiji. A high proportion of the selected Australian soft drink manufacturers (60%) and fast food restaurants (80%) had policies available online, whereas this was the case for only a small minority of companies in these sectors in New Zealand and Fiji.

The selected companies were signatories to a number of national and global industry initiatives related to product formulation. In Australia, these included the Healthy Australia Commitment (Australian Food and Grocery Council, 2012) (seven of the eight signatories to the Healthy Australian Commitment are included in the selected companies for Australia) and the commitments of the Australian Beverages Council (Australian Beverages Council, 2014). In New Zealand, four of the selected companies were part of the HeartSafe initiative aimed at sodium and saturated fat reduction (the latter only for savoury pies) (Heart Foundation, 2014). None of the selected New Zealand companies were members of The Chip Group, a New Zealand initiative that sets standards related to portion size, oil use (*trans* and saturated fat standards) and addition of salt for outlets serving chips (The Chip Group, 2014). In Fiji, all of the selected soft drink manufacturers were signatories to a Memorandum of Understanding that includes a product formulation component (Fiji Beverages Group, 2014). These initiatives were in addition to product formulation commitments many of the selected companies have made through the IFBA (International Food and Beverage Alliance, 2014).

Across all three countries, the highest proportion of product formulation policies included salt reduction and product portfolio changes (for example, aiming to include a higher proportion of healthier products in their product mix). Fewer policies focused on fat, including saturated fat and/or *trans* fat, reduction. Very few of the selected companies had policies on added sugar and energy reduction. Refer to Table 4 for further details.

As with the policies related to food marketing to children, the seven companies that were included in the selection for all three countries each maintained largely consistent policies across Australia, New Zealand and Fiji.

Discussion

This analysis has shown that there are important differences in the prevalence of publicly available policies relating to food marketing to children and product formulation amongst the most prominent food companies in Australia, New Zealand and Fiji. In Australia and New Zealand, there were a higher proportion of companies with publicly available policies than in Fiji. However, even in Australia and New Zealand, there were a large proportion of the most prominent food companies that did not have publicly available policies in these domains. In Australia, there was a high prevalence of industry initiatives with respect to food marketing to children and product formulation, but these were less prevalent in New Zealand and Fiji. Where they existed, policies on food marketing to children generally focused on those aged less than 12, did not apply to all types of media, marketing channels and techniques, and did not provide transparency with respect to the products to which the policies apply. Product formulation policies, where they existed, tended to focus on salt reduction and changes to the make-up of overall product portfolios, and did not generally address saturated fat, added sugar and energy reduction. This study found that, for the most part, the policies of multinational companies were consistent across the three countries. However, it was often difficult to ascertain exactly what a company's policy in a particular area was, due to a lack of clear and transparent disclosure.

This paper is the first to provide an assessment of the policies of food companies in the Pacific region with respect to food marketing to children and product formulation. However, the findings of this paper are generally consistent with previous efforts to assess the policies of food companies in these domains at a global level (Access to Nutrition Index, 2013; Lang, Rayner, & Kaelin, 2006). These previous studies also found substantial differences in the nature of the policies and the level of disclosure and transparency amongst different companies. When the policies of the companies investigated in this study are compared to the recommendations for the private sector by leading international and national health organisations (refer to Table 1), it is apparent that a substantial proportion of the companies investigated are either not taking the recommended actions or not making their actions publicly available. However, it is also acknowledged that many of the recommended actions for the private sector outlined in Table 1 are non-specific, and do not provide detailed guidance on what should be included in a company policy. For example, the IOM recommends that the private sector shift their product portfolio to foods that are lower in total energy, fats, salts and added sugars and have a higher positive nutrient content (Institute of Medicine, 2006). This recommendation, similar to that from other organisations, does not provide specific limits or targets for which companies should be aiming. Nevertheless, the WHO guidelines were used to underpin other industry schemes, such as the Health and Wellness Initiative of The Consumer Good Forum (The Consumer Goods Forum, 2013).

There are currently no globally agreed benchmarks against which to compare the content of company policies related to food marketing and product formulation, although ATNI provides performance criteria against a number of relevant indicators with respect to food and beverage manufacturers (Access to Nutrition Index, 2013). While it was beyond the scope of this study to perform a detailed assessment of each company's policies, future studies in Australia, New Zealand and Fiji could adapt the ATNI criteria for this purpose. In addition, researchers should aim to identify particular companies that can be held up as exemplars of good practice. For example, it would appear that Unilever applies their product formulation policy across all the countries in which they operate (Unilever, 2014); however, the extent to which this is implemented is currently unclear.

This study has several limitations. Firstly, data collection included only content that was available online. Companies were not contacted directly to provide information about their policies or to verify the data collected, and so it is possible that companies have publicly available policies that were not included in the analysis. In Fiji, in particular, many of the selected companies did not have a company website. Future studies should seek to involve companies as part of the data collection process. Secondly, this study did not investigate the extent to which companies have implemented their policies or their actual performance with respect to food marketing to children and product formulation. These aspects will be investigated as part of the 'expanded' and 'optimal' steps of the private sector module of INFORMAS (Sacks et al., 2013), or as part of future phases of ATNI (Access to Nutrition Index, 2013). Thirdly, while this study assessed three different sectors of the food industry, it did not further distinguish between industry sub-sectors, such as dairy. Furthermore, it did not distinguish between company characteristics such as ownership structure, financial position, size, culture, product portfolio and readiness for change. Future studies should investigate how these characteristics influence the degree to which companies are able to comply with public health recommendations, and take leadership positions within the industry. For example, it appears from the analysis conducted in this study that dairy companies and supermarkets are less likely to have policies in the area of food marketing to children and product formulation, but this needs further investigation. Fourthly, this study focused on the most prominent food companies in each country. There is a risk that, in doing so, we fail to recognise the practices of less prominent companies, and we may also serve to promote the interests of the larger companies. However, it is the larger companies that are in a position to influence the industry culture, and they have greater influence on government policies. Future studies should seek to identify good practice examples from across the food industry, whilst also monitoring food company practices that undermine health (Sacks et al., 2013). Finally, the focus on private sector policies independent of public sector policies in each domain may limit the extent to which cross-country comparisons are meaningful. As part of INFORMAS, future monitoring efforts will focus on both public and private sector policies and actions (Swinburn et al., 2013). More broadly, this paper did not analyse political, economic, social and technological factors that may influence differences in company policies across countries.

Conclusions

This analysis has shown that there are large differences in the prevalence of company food marketing and product formulation policies between high-income countries, such as Australia and New Zealand, and a middle-income country, such as Fiji. Even in Australia, where there are highly active industry associations and strong pressure from public-interest groups for companies to take action, a large proportion of the most prominent food companies do not have publicly available policies related to food marketing to children and product formulation. In the absence of strong policies and corresponding actions by the private sector, it is likely that government action (e.g. through co-regulation or legislation) will be needed to drive improved company performance.

In consideration of the severity of the obesity and diet-related NCDs problem globally, and the recognition of the important role of the food industry in being part of the problems and solutions, there is an imperative for major food companies to be publicly accountable for their actions to improve the healthiness of food environments. Food companies are increasingly expected to make public their policies and commitments regarding food marketing to children and product formulation, and to apply these policies and commitments consistently across locations. Accordingly, the monitoring of private sector nutrition policies is just the beginning. Where food companies have publicly available policies, the next step is to hold them to account for their performance in relation to their policies, and aim to improve their policies with reference to global benchmarks.

Acknowledgements

This work was supported by the Australian National Health and Medical Research Council under Grant APP1041020. The authors wish to acknowledge Amy Xiao for her assistance with data collection for New Zealand, and Lennart Sick for his assistance with preliminary data collection for Australia. Thanks also to Arti Pillay, Astika Raj, Arleen Sukhu, Jillian Wate from the C-POND team for their input into the selection of companies in Fiji. The authors declare that they have no competing interests.

References

Access to Nutrition Index. (2013). Access to nutrition index: Global index 2013. Retrieved March 2014, from http://www.accesstonutrition.org

Advertising Standards Authority. (2010). Children's code for advertising food 2010. Retrieved March 2014, from http://www.asa.co.nz/code_children_food.php

Australian Association of National Advertisers. (2013). Code for advertising and marketing communications to children. Retrieved March 2014, from http://www.aana.com.au/codes/AANA_Code_of_Advertising_Marketing_Comms_to_Children_FINAL.pdf

Australian Beverages Council. (2014). Marketing to children. Retrieved March 2014, from http://australianbeverages.org/for-consumers/marketing-to-children/

Australian Food and Grocery Council. (1995). Code of practice on nutrient claims in food labels and in advertisements. Retrieved March 2014, from http://www.foodstandards.gov.au/publications/documents/Code_of_Practice_jan1995.pdf

Australian Food and Grocery Council. (2012). Healthier Australia Commitment. Food and Beverage Innovation. Aiming to improve the health of Australian families. Retrieved March 2014, from http://www.togethercounts.com.au/wp-content/uploads/2013/02/HAC-Food-Targets.pdf

Australian Food and Grocery Council. (2014a). Quick service restaurant initiative for responsible advertising and marketing to children. Updated January 2014. Retrieved March 2014, from http://www.afgc.org.au/health-and-nutrition/industry-codes/advertising-to-children/qsr-initiative.html

Australian Food and Grocery Council. (2014b). Responsible children's marketing initiative. Updated January 2014. Retrieved March 2014, from http://www.afgc.org.au/doc-library/category/11-general-documents.html?download=1001%3Aupdated-rcmi-1-january-2014

Brinsden, H., Lobstein, T., Landon, J., Kraak, V., Sacks, G., Kumanyika, S., … Walker, C. (2013). Monitoring policy and actions on food environments: Rationale and outline of the INFORMAS policy engagement and communication strategies. *Review of Obesity Reviews, 14*, 13–23. doi:10.1111/obr.12072

Brownell, K. D., & Horgen, K. B. (2004). *Food fight: The inside story of the food industry, America's obesity crisis and what we can do about it.* Chicago, IL: Contemporary Books.

Brownell, K. D., & Warner, K. E. (2009). The perils of ignoring history: Big Tobacco played dirty and millions died. How similar is Big Food? *Milbank Quarterly, 87*, 259–294. doi: MILQ555 [pii] 10.1111/j.1468-0009.2009.00555.x

Elliott, T., Trevena, H., Sacks, G., Dunford, E., Martin, J., Webster, J., … Neal, B. C. (2014). A systematic interim assessment of the Australian Government's Food and Health Dialogue. *The Medical Journal of Australia, 200*, 92–95.

Euromonitor International. (2013). Passport. Retrieved March 2014, from http://www.euromonitor.com/passport

Fiji Beverages Group. (2014). Memorandum of understanding – Supporting healthy active lives for people in Fiji. Retrieved March 2014, from http://fijibeveragegroup.theclique.co.nz/memorandumofunderstanding/

Gortmaker, S. L., Swinburn, B. A., Levy, D., Carter, R., Mabry, P. L., Finegood, D. T., … Moodie, M. L. (2011). Changing the future of obesity: Science, policy, and action. *The Lancet, 378*, 838–847. doi:S0140-6736(11)60815-5 [pii] 10.1016/S0140-6736(11)60815-5

Heart Foundation. (2014). HeartSAFE. Retrieved March 2014, from http://www.heartfoundation.org.nz/programmes-resources/food-industry-and-hospitality/heartsafe

Institute of Medicine. (2006). *Food marketing to children: Threat or opportunity?* Washington, DC: National Academies Press.

International Association for the Study of Obesity. (2010). The PolMark Project – Policies on marketing food and beverages to children. Final project report Annex 1. Retrieved March 2014, from http://www.worldobesity.org/site_media/uploads/The_PolMark_Project_Final_Report_Annex_1_FINAL.pdf

International Council of Beverages Associations. (2012). International Council of Beverages Associations, Guidelines on marketing to children. Retrieved March 2014, from http://www. icba-net.org/files/resources/icba-marketing-to-children-guidelines.pdf

International Food and Beverage Alliance. (2011). Global policy on advertising and marketing communications to children, November 2011. Retrieved March 2014, from https://www.ifbal liance.org/sites/default/files/IFBAGlobalPolicyonAdvertisingandMarketingCommunicationsto ChildrenFINAL112011.pdf

International Food and Beverage Alliance. (2014). Product composition and availability. Retrieved March 2014, from https://ifballiance.org/our-commitments/commitment-1-product-composition -and-availability/

Lang, T., Rayner, G., & Kaelin, E. (2006). *The food industry, diet, physical activity and health: A review of reported commitments and practice of 25 of the world's largest food companies.* London: City University. Retrieved from http://www.city.ac.uk/news/press/The%20Food% 20Industry%20Diet%20Physical%20Activity%20and%20Health.pdf

Lumley, J., Martin, J., & Antonopoulos, N. (2012). *Exposing the Charade – The failure to protect children from unhealthy food advertising.* Melbourne: Obesity Policy Coalition. Retrieved from http://www.opc.org.au/downloads/OPC_Exposing_the_Charade_report_2012.pdf

Ministry of Health. (2007). *National Nutrition Survey.* Suva: Ministry of Health.

Monteiro, C. A., Gomes, F. S., & Cannon, G. (2010). The snack attack. *American Journal of Public Health, 100*, 975–981. doi:10.2105/AJPH.2009.187666

Moodie, R., Stuckler, D., Monteiro, C., Sheron, N., Neal, B., Thamarangsi, T., … N.C.D. Action Group Lancet. (2013). Profits and pandemics: Prevention of harmful effects of tobacco, alco- hol, and ultra-processed food and drink industries. *The Lancet, 381*, 670–679. doi:10.1016/ S0140-6736(12)62089-3

Neal, B., Sacks, G., Swinburn, B., Vandevijvere, S., Dunford, E., Snowdon, W., … Walker, C. (2013). Monitoring the levels of important nutrients in the food supply. *Obesity Reviews, 14*, 49–58. doi:10.1111/obr.12075

Nestle, M. (2002). *Food politics: How the Food industry influences nutrition and health.* Los Angeles: University of California Press.

Nestle. (2014a). Responsible advertising & marketing. Retrieved March 2014, from http://www. nestle.com.au/aboutus/nestle-the-company/responsible-advertising–marketing

Nestle. (2014b). Responsible advertising and marketing. Retrieved March 2014, from http://www. nestle.com/csv/human-rights-compliance/advertising-marketing

Sacks, G., Swinburn, B., Kraak, V., Downs, S., Walker, C., Barquera, S., … Walker, C. (2013). A proposed approach to monitor private-sector policies and practices related to food environ- ments, obesity and non-communicable disease prevention. *Obesity Reviews, 14*, 38–48. doi:10.1111/obr.12074

Snowdon, W., Raj, A., Reeve, E., Guerrero, R., Fesaitu, J., Cateine, K., & Guignet, C. (2013). Processed foods available in the Pacific Islands. *Globalization and Health, 9*, 53. doi:10.1186/1744-8603-9-53

Swinburn, B., Sacks, G., Vandevijvere, S., Kumanyika, S., Lobstein, T., Neal, B., … Walker, C. (2013). INFORMAS (International Network for Food and Obesity/non-communicable diseases Research, Monitoring and Action Support): Overview and key principles. *Obesity Reviews, 14*(Suppl 1), 1–12. doi:10.1111/obr.12087

The Chip Group. (2014). The Chip Group. Retrieved March 2014, from http://blog.thechipgroup. co.nz/the-chip-group-2/

The Consumer Goods Forum. (2013). Health and wellness resolutions, progress report, co- authored by Deloitte. Retrieved March 2014, from http://tcgfhealthandwellness.com/measure ment-a-reporting/measurement-and-reporting-report-health-and-wellness.html

The PLoS Medicine Editors. (2012). PLoS medicine series on big food: The food industry is ripe for scrutiny. *PLoS Medicine, 9*, 1–2. doi:10.1371/journal.pmed.1001246

Unilever. (2014). Sustainable living: Improving nutrition – Targets and performance. Retrieved March 2014, from http://www.unilever.com/sustainable-living/nutrition-health/targetsandperformance/

United Nations. (2011). *Political declaration of the high-level meeting of the general assembly on the prevention and control of non-communicable diseases*. New York, NY: United Nations, General Assembly.

World Cancer Research Fund/American Institute for Cancer Research. (2009). Policy and action for cancer prevention. Food, nutrition, physical activity, and the prevention of cancer: A global perspective. Washington, DC: American Institute for Cancer Research.

World Health Organization. (2004). *Global strategy on diet, physical activity and health*. Geneva: Author.

World Health Organization. (2010). *Set of recommendations on the marketing of foods and non-alcoholic beverages to children*. Geneva: Author.

World Health Organization. (2011). Global status report on noncommunicable diseases 2010. Geneva: Author.

World Health Organization. (2013). *Global action plan for the prevention and control of non-communicable diseases 2013–2020*. Geneva: Author.

Yale Rudd Center for Food Policy and Obesity. (2014). Marketing pledges. Retrieved March 2014, from http://www.yaleruddcenter.org/marketingpledges

Encouraging big food to do the right thing for children's health: a case study on using research to improve marketing of sugary cereals

Jennifer L. Harris, Megan E. LoDolce and Marlene B. Schwartz

Rudd Center for Food Policy and Obesity, Yale University, New Haven, CT, USA

Addressing concerns about unhealthy food marketing to children, food companies pledge to advertise only 'healthier dietary choices' in 'child-directed media'. However, public health advocates question whether the food industry will voluntarily improve their child-targeted marketing practices in a meaningful way. In this paper, we evaluate progress made by manufacturers of one food category – ready-to-eat breakfast cereals – in promoting nutritious choices to children, and the potential role of scientific research to influence corporate behavior. Beginning in 2008, researchers at the Rudd Center for Food Policy & Obesity conducted a series of studies to evaluate child-targeted marketing by cereal companies using a variety of research methods. We aimed to understand the extent and impact of cereal marketing to children; disseminate these findings to parents, the media, the public health community, policy-makers, and industry representatives; and encourage cereal companies to shift child-targeted marketing toward the more nutritious products in their portfolios. A follow-up analysis in 2012 demonstrated some improvements in the nutritional quality and marketing of child-targeted cereals, although child-targeted cereals remain the least healthy products in company portfolios. This analysis provides a case study of the potential for success, as well as the limitations, of a public health strategy to incent food companies to voluntarily improve child-targeted marketing practices through strategic research and communications.

Introduction

Numerous environmental factors have likely fueled the dramatic rise in childhood obesity and contributed to poor diets among young people in the United States. Public health experts point to the overwhelming amount of marketing for unhealthy foods and beverages targeted to children as a significant influence (Institute of Medicine [IOM], 2006). Products most commonly marketed to children contain high levels of saturated fat, added sugars, and sodium that can lead to obesity and diet-related diseases such as type 2 diabetes and heart disease (Federal Trade Commission [FTC], 2012; Powell, Schermbeck, Szczypka, Chaloupka, & Braunschweig, 2011). Exposure to unhealthy food marketing also negatively impacts children's food preferences, consumption of unhealthy categories of foods, and total calories consumed (White House Task Force on Childhood Obesity, 2010).

Responding to growing concerns about unhealthy food marketing to children and the food and beverage industry's role in the obesity crisis, in 2006, the Council of Better Business Bureaus launched an industry self-regulatory program, the Children's Food and Beverage Advertising Initiative (CFBAI) (Kolish & Enright, 2013). Through this initiative, 17 major food and beverage companies pledge to only advertise 'healthier dietary choices' in 'child-directed media'. The goal is to 'shift the mix of advertising messages directed to children under 12 to encourage healthier dietary choices and lifestyles'.

Despite companies' CFBAI pledges, independent reviews conducted in recent years have found limited improvements in food marketing to children. For example, youth-targeted food marketing expenditures declined from $2.1 billion in 2006 to $1.8 billion in 2009 (FTC, 2012). However, closer analysis reveals that two-thirds of this decline was due to reductions in fast-food kids' meal premiums and advertising on children's television; while less expensive forms of marketing, including digital media, sponsorships, product placements, and philanthropic promotions increased (Powell, Harris, & Fox, 2013). Furthermore, improvements in the nutritional quality of products advertised to children have been small and slow. For example, in 2009, 86% of food-related TV advertisements viewed by children promoted products high in saturated fat, sugar, or sodium, compared with 94% in 2003 (Powell et al., 2011). In 2013, First Lady Michelle Obama urged food companies, 'to do even more and move even faster to market responsibly to our kids'. (The White House, 2013).

In this paper, we evaluate the progress by manufacturers of one food category – ready-to-eat breakfast cereals – to promote nutritious choices to children. We demonstrate the role that scientific research together with communication of findings to audiences whose actions could affect cereal-company profits (including parents, the media, and policy-makers) can play in influencing corporate behavior. This analysis provides a case study in the potential for success, as well as the limitations, of a public health strategy to incent food companies to voluntarily improve child-targeted marketing practices.

Why children's cereals?

Beginning in 2008, researchers at the Rudd Center for Food Policy & Obesity conducted a series of studies in the United States to evaluate child-targeted marketing by cereal companies. We focused on children's cereals because they represented the packaged-food category marketed most often to children on TV (Powell, Szczypka, & Chaloupka, 2007) and the internet (Alvy & Calvert, 2008). In 2006, cereal companies spent $229 million on all forms of marketing directly targeting children under 12, more than any other food category (FTC, 2008). Furthermore, child-targeted cereals (defined as brands with one or more of the following on the package: a licensed character, television, movie theme; any other cartoon drawing; a promotion that was directed at children) consisted of 32–43% sugar by weight and were less nutritious than other cereal products (Schwartz, Vartanian, Wharton, & Brownell, 2008). Thus, companies could switch child-targeted marketing toward existing more nutritious products without expensive and time-consuming reformulations (potential barriers to improving child-targeted marketing). Finally, only four companies advertised cereals to children (General Mills, Kellogg, Post, & Quaker) (Schwartz et al., 2010), and all belong to the CFBAI (Kolish & Enright, 2013). Therefore, cereal companies pledged to improve their marketing to children, providing an opportunity to examine whether company actions complied with publicly stated intentions.

Importantly, we also identified an opportunity to address public misconceptions about benefits of serving high-sugar cereals to children. Research funded by cereal companies demonstrated health benefits of consuming cereals versus skipping breakfast altogether (Albertson et al., 2009) or versus consuming high-fat options, such as fried eggs and bacon (Cho, Dietrich, Brown, Clark, & Block, 2003), and the US Department of Agriculture (USDA, 2010) recommends that children consume cereal, together with milk and fruit, as components of a healthy breakfast. However, research had not compared differences between consuming child-targeted (i.e. high sugar) and low-sugar cereals (Castetbon, Harris, & Schwartz, 2012). Furthermore, despite growing concerns about sugar consumption (Johnson et al., 2009), cereal companies claimed that children will not eat low-sugar cereals (Clark & Crockett, 2008), and these products provide valuable micronutrients (e.g. vitamin D, calcium) (Thompson, Franko, & Barton, 2008).

Strategic science approach

Thus, existing research demonstrated that cereal companies aggressively market high-sugar cereals directly to children; companies may misinform parents and the public about the benefits of serving high-sugar cereals to children; and the CFBAI industry self-regulatory program may not effectively limit unhealthy cereal marketing to children. To evaluate these potential public-health issues, we conducted strategic research studies to better understand cereal companies' child-directed marketing practices and how they affect children. We aimed to identify opportunities for cereal companies to improve child-targeted marketing practices and communicate our findings to audiences whose actions could affect cereal companies' sales and profits. These key change agents included parents who buy the cereals, policy-makers who could enact regulation or legislation to govern cereal-company actions, the media and advocates who could help inform parents and encourage policy-makers to act, and the cereal manufacturers themselves.

To identify the key research questions, we considered potential reasons why parents buy high-sugar cereals and why they were not more concerned about child-targeted food marketing. We conducted focus groups (Ustjanauskas et al., 2010), followed by a large survey of parents (Speers, Goren, Harris, Schwartz, & Brownell, 2009), to understand parents' perceptions about food marketing to their children. We learned that parents were largely unaware of all the ways that food companies market unhealthy foods to children, especially marketing on the internet. However, they became outraged when informed about common online child-targeted marketing practices, such as advergames (i.e. branded food-company games). In addition, quantitative analyses revealed that understanding the extent of child-targeted marketing was not sufficient to increase support for food-marketing restrictions; parents also must understand how this marketing affects their children (Goren, Harris, Schwartz, & Brownell, 2010). Therefore, an important research goal was to document how cereal companies market to children, especially on the internet, and to demonstrate the impact of marketing on children's diets and health.

We also considered cereal-company marketing practices that might raise the policy-maker concerns. We hypothesized that the promotion of high-sugar cereals as nutritious options for children could mislead consumers and justify policy action, including common industry practices of adding micronutrients to otherwise nutrient-poor products and identifying high-sugar cereals as 'healthier dietary choices' through the CFBAI. In addition, cereal companies had identified many nutritionally poor children's cereals as 'Smart Choices', using criteria developed by the food industry to qualify for a front-of-pack label identifying healthier products (Smart Choices, 2009). Therefore, another research goal was to evaluate the overall nutritional quality of children's cereals and determine whether messages promoting high-sugar cereals as healthier choices misled consumers into thinking these products were nutritious options for children.

Finally, we examined cereal-company statements defending their marketing practices to identify potential industry counterarguments. In response to previous studies documenting high-sugar content in children's cereals, companies claimed that children would not eat low-sugar cereals. In a letter to the editor of the *Journal of the American Dietetic Association*, nutritionists from Kellogg and General Mills stated, 'Food does not become nutrition until it is eaten', and 'Children like the taste of ready-to-eat cereals and are therefore more likely to eat breakfast' (Clark & Crockett, 2008). However, research had not confirmed this strategy for improving children's diets, presenting an opportunity to empirically test this claim.

As an academic research center, we are committed to transparency and utilizing the best scientific practices. We value peer-reviewed academic research, but studies published in academic journals often are outdated by the time of publication, making them less useful for current policy work. Furthermore, strict word requirements can limit the amount of specific and detailed information we could present about cereal-company marketing practices. Therefore, we designed all research to meet the standards for scientific journals to maintain the credibility of the findings, but supplemented academic papers with timely self-published reports that detailed specific company and brand-level information for use by advocates and policy-makers.

The research

From 2008 to 2012, researchers at the Rudd Center conducted several studies to document cereal nutrition, marketing targeted to children, and effects on children and their parents. Our 2009 report, *Cereal FACTS: Evaluating the Nutrition Quality and Marketing of Children's Cereals* (Harris et al., 2009) served as the cornerstone of this research program. It provided a comprehensive and science-based evaluation of cereal marketing to children, including on TV, the internet, and in stores, following implementation of companies' CFBAI pledges. It also compared the nutritional quality of cereals marketed to children with adult-targeted cereals. The report utilized syndicated market research data, supplemented by in-house and commissioned studies when the data were not publicly available. Additional studies examined the extent and impact of specific practices identified in *Cereal FACTS*.

Documenting cereal nutrition and child-targeted marketing

Results of *Cereal FACTS* demonstrated that the CFBAI had not led to noticeable improvements in child-targeted cereal marketing (Harris et al., 2009). In 2009, sugar content of child-targeted cereals averaged three teaspoons per serving (approximately one-third of cereal content by weight), down from 3.5 teaspoons in 2006. In addition, child-targeted cereals contained 85% more sugar, 60% more sodium, and 65% less fiber than cereals targeted to adults. Products with the worst nutrition ratings (e.g. *Reeses' Puffs*, *Corn Pops*, *Lucky Charms*) were deemed 'better-for-you' in companies' CFBAI pledges and the industry's Smart Choices front-of-pack labeling program. Not one CFBAI-approved cereal qualified for the USDA Women, Infants and Children (WIC) program, and none would be allowed in advertising to children in the United Kingdom. We identified a category of 'family cereals' (e.g. plain *Cheerios, Frosted Mini-Wheats, Life*) that were more nutritious than child-targeted cereals, but companies chose to market these products exclusively to parents, not children. We also highlighted the common practice of placing nutrition-related claims on unhealthy cereals: 95% of child-targeted cereal boxes displayed at least one nutrition-related claim (e.g. contains whole grains, vitamin D, and calcium), while many featured three to four such claims.

Furthermore, in 2008–2009, companies continued to aggressively advertise their least nutritious cereals to children on television and the internet (Harris et al., 2009). On average, children viewed 1.6 advertisements per day on television promoting high-sugar children's cereals. Eight child-targeted advergame sites featured high-sugar cereals on most pages and typically incorporated the cereal as part of the game (e.g. creating bumper boats out of *Fruity Cheerios* or brand characters in an *Apple Jacks* racing game). The two most popular sites, Millsberry.com and Postopia.com, averaged 767,000 and 265,000 young visitors per month, respectively. Millsberry was especially engaging, featuring a virtual world where children could create their own avatar and explore a branded 'city'. Visitors averaged 66 min per month on the site. In addition, cereal companies placed banner advertising on popular children's websites (e.g. Nick.com, Disney Channel) to drive traffic to their advergames. In the supermarket, 21% of the cereal aisle was devoted to child-targeted cereals, and special displays were more likely to feature child-targeted cereals compared with adult cereals. Furthermore, product packaging featured numerous messages to attract children's attention, such as promotions and brand characters on the front and games and advergame URLs on the back.

Two additional studies further documented the extent of cereal-company marketing targeted to children. Using syndicated market research data from comScore, we analyzed child visitors to all food company websites and found that websites containing advergames attracted twice as many children compared with other sites (Harris, Speers, Schwartz, & Brownell, 2012). Advergame sites also were more engaging, and cereal companies maintained the most popular advergame sites (Harris, Weinberg, Javadizadeh, & Sarda, 2013). In the supermarket, cereal companies also were more likely to use child-targeted promotions than other food companies, which featured on 19% of cereal boxes (Harris, Schwartz, & Brownell, 2010). Two cereal companies (Kellogg and General Mills) had more child-targeted cross-promotions than any other food manufacturer. Furthermore, from 2006 to 2008 (pre- and post-CFBAI implementation), promotions in the supermarket increased, especially those targeting preschoolers and older youth, but the nutritional quality of promoted products did not improve.

Effects of child-targeted cereal marketing

We also assessed the impact of advergames, nutrition-related claims on high-sugar cereals, and messages used to promote high-sugar cereals to children. In an experiment examining the effects of playing advergames on children's snacking behavior, children ages 7–12 were randomly assigned to play advergames promoting unhealthy foods, advergames promoting healthy foods, or control games without food mentions (Harris, Speers et al., 2012). After playing, researchers offered children a variety of healthy and unhealthy snacks. Playing unhealthy advergames increased children's consumption of unhealthy snack foods by 56% and reduced fruits and vegetables consumption by one-third. Furthermore, effects were greater for children who regularly played advergames, suggesting that repeated exposure increases advertising effectiveness.

We also examined how parents interpreted nutrition-related claims on high-sugar cereal packages in an online survey of parents (Harris, Thompson, Schwartz, & Brownell, 2011). Parents misinterpreted claims that highlighted specific nutrients, such as whole grain or fiber, and other more general claims (e.g. 'supports your child's immunity'), believing that nutritionally poor cereals with these claims were more nutritious than other cereals. Claims also increased parents' willingness to buy. Parents also inferred incorrect information about claim meaning, including that they provided health benefits that the FDA does not allow companies to state directly. For example, 80% of parents assumed that cereals with 'calcium and Vitamin D' would help their child grow strong bones, and 74% believed that cereals with 'antioxidants and vitamins' would keep their child from getting sick. Thus, nutrition-related claims potentially misled consumers about the true nutritional quality and potential health benefits of child-targeted cereals.

We also content analyzed the messages in television advertisements for high-sugar cereals and measured children's exposure to those advertisements using Nielsen data (LoDolce, Harris, & Schwartz, 2013). Nearly all (87%) cereal advertisements seen by children promoted high-sugar products, whereas adults were equally likely to see adver-tisements for high- and low-sugar cereals. In addition, messages in high-sugar cereal advertisements that children viewed were significantly more likely to convey unrealistic messages and misleading information about healthy eating. For example, 91% portrayed cereals as having extraordinary powers (e.g. cereal pieces transforming into cartoon characters, roller coasters, and playthings), and 67% portrayed both healthy and unhealthy behaviors in the same ad (e.g. eating at non-meal times, indicating the cereal is part of a balanced breakfast). These unrealistic, highly entertaining, and mixed mes-sages raise concerns given children's greater vulnerability to advertising influence and limited ability to evaluate advertising truthfulness (IOM, 2006).

Potential cereal-company responses

We also conducted an experiment to test cereal companies' claim that children will only eat high-sugar cereals (Harris, Schwartz, Ustjanauskas, Ohri-Vachaspati, & Brownell, 2011). Children were randomly assigned to choose one of three high-sugar or compara-ble low-sugar cereals (e.g. *Frosted Flakes* vs. *Corn Flakes*) for breakfast served in sum-mer day camps. Participants in both groups also served themselves low-fat milk, orange juice, bananas, and strawberries. Sugar packets were provided in both conditions. All children reported either 'liking' or 'loving' the cereal they chose, with no difference between those who received high- vs. low-sugar cereals. Children ate significantly more high-sugar cereals (two servings vs. approximately one in the low-sugar group). Nota-bly, although children added more table sugar to low-sugar cereals, children in the high-sugar condition consumed almost twice as much refined sugar overall due to the sugar in the presweetened cereals. Milk and total calories consumed did not differ sig-nificantly between groups, but children in the low-sugar condition ate more fruit. There-fore, children who were offered low-sugar cereals had a more nutritious breakfast overall.

Finally, we examined cereal-purchasing patterns using Nielsen Homescan data to assess the relationship between purchasing behavior, nutritional quality, marketing strategy, and household socio-demographic characteristics (Castetbon et al., 2012). Households with at least one child purchased the most cereals. Households with children, as well as African–American and Hispanic households, purchased more unhealthy cereals compared with other households. In addition, households purchased child-targeted cereals with advertising 13 times more often than non-advertised brands, while advertised adult cereals were purchased four times as often. These results suggest that advertising to children is more effective than advertising to adults and leads to greater consumption of nutritionally poor products, especially in households with children.

Communicating the research findings

Communications represented an integral component of our public health strategy to encourage companies to improve their marketing to children. The release of *Cereal FACTS* in late 2009 was accompanied by extensive communications targeting three key change agents: parents (i.e. cereal-company customers), advocates, policy-makers, and other researchers. We created a website (CerealFACTS.org) featuring consumer-friendly information for parents and advocates, including interactive tools to evaluate the nutritional quality of different brands and identify healthier choices, and rankings of brands by the type of marketing. We also created a four-page summary of the report for distribution to press and policy-makers. In the accompanying public relations campaign, we focused on one primary message: 'Cereal companies aggressively market their least nutritious products directly to children', requesting that companies, 'Market the more nutritious products that are already in their portfolios instead of high-sugar cereals to children'. Further, we conducted outreach to state and national policy-makers.

The results were news. *Cereal FACTS* received over 400 mentions in national and local TV, radio, and print, and the coverage was overwhelmingly positive (Yale Rudd Center, 2014). The media also addressed the common misperception that high-sugar cereals are healthy options for children's breakfast. In subsequent years, we published the follow-up studies in academic journals, which also received widespread national media attention. In addition, CerealFACTS.org received over 136,000 visits. The industry responded quickly. Shortly after the report's publication, General Mills launched its own website and public relations campaign defending its products and marketing practices (General Mills, 2014). General Mills and Post both announced further added-sugar reductions in their children's cereals (NBC News, 2010; Skidmore, 2009). PepsiCo took down its child-targeted *Cap'n Crunch* website (*Crunch Island*). Finally, three of the four major cereal companies agreed to meet with us to discuss opportunities to improve marketing to children.

Policy-makers also paid attention. The release of *Cereal FACTS* coincided with industry's announcement of its new Smart Choices labeling program (Smart Choices, 2009). The combination of our report and a *NY Times* article questioning whether *Froot Loops* should be a Smart Choice (Neuman, 2009) caught the attention of Connecticut's Attorney General Richard Blumenthal. Mr Blumenthal announced that the Smart Choices program was 'potentially misleading' and initiated an investigation. One week later, the FDA announced that it also would analyze 'misleading' food labels and nutrition standards (without naming Smart Choices directly). On 23rd October, Smart Choices was officially put on hold pending the FDA's findings (Ruiz, 2009).

Evaluating industry promises

The CFBAI's annual report for 2012 cited substantial progress in food and beverage marketing to children since the Initiative's inception in 2006, 'The work that the CFBAI's participants have done to change the children's food advertising landscape shows that strong, thoughtful and transparent self-regulation can make an important difference' (Kolish & Enright, 2013). The report highlights companies' excellent compliance with their pledges; the enhanced nutritional content of foods advertised to children and the introduction of new category-specific uniform nutrition standards to be implemented by 2014; and the Initiative's expansion to additional food manufacturers and one media company. The report notes that the positive trend in nutrition 'was particularly notable in the cereal category'.

However, continued independent evaluation of food-marketing practices is necessary to determine whether meaningful change has occurred. Thus in 2012, we issued an update on the original *Cereal FACTS* report using the same methods and data sources as the 2009 report (Harris, Schwartz et al., 2012). This report measured changes in cereal nutrition and marketing targeted to children during the intervening three years.

In *Cereal FACTS 2012*, we identified several positive developments. Overall nutritional quality improved for 13 of the 16 child-targeted brands, by 10% on average. General Mills and Post discontinued their popular advergame sites (Millsberry.com and Postopia.com), resulting in an estimated 31% fewer internet advertisements viewed by children. On television, children viewed 5% fewer cereal advertisements in 2011 than in 2008 and 23% fewer vs. 2006. By comparison, children's exposure to TV advertisements for most other packaged-food categories increased from 2008 to 2011. For example, candy advertising to children was more than doubled and advertisements for all other packaged foods and beverages increased by 6%.

On the other hand, some findings were less encouraging. Total media spending for child-targeted cereals increased by 34%; children's exposure to TV advertising increased by 25% or more for some high-sugar cereals (*Froot Loops, Reese's Puffs, Trix,* and *Pebbles*); Post and General Mills launched new smaller advergame websites for some child-targeted brands; and banner advertising and child visitors increased for most child-targeted websites that existed in 2008 and 2011. Kellogg also introduced the first cereal-company child-targeted advergame mobile app and a new high-sugar cereal (*Krave*) targeted to 12–14-year-olds.

Thus, there was some progress from 2008 to 2011, as well as evidence of new concerns. However, cereal companies' overall strategy for marketing to children did not change substantially. In 2011, as in 2008, they continued to market their worst products directly to children. Despite improvements, cereals advertised to children contained 57% more sugar, 50% more sodium, and 52% less fiber than adult-targeted cereals; while parents remained the primary target for more nutritious 'family' cereals (e.g. *Frosted Mini-Wheats, Multigrain Cheerios*). Children continued to see more advertisements on television for cereals than any other packaged-food category (almost two advertisements per day). Finally, the majority of cereal advertisements seen by children on television promoted products consisting of one-third or more sugar. We found no evidence that companies had begun to market healthier products directly to children. Only Quaker had stopped advertising to children directly, repositioning its *Cap'n Crunch* cereal to adults with a nostalgia positioning.

Discussion

Rudd Center research on ready-to-eat breakfast cereals marketed in the United States was part of a national effort by researchers and advocacy groups to highlight the poor nutritional quality of children's cereals and aggressive marketing practices targeting children (e.g. Kunkel, McKinley, & Wright, 2009; Powell et al., 2011). Government initiatives also have raised public awareness of unhealthy food marketing to children, including First Lady Michelle Obama's White House Task Force (2010) report on food marketing to children, two FTC (2008, 2012) reports on marketing expenditures targeted to children and adolescents, and an Interagency Working Group on Food Marketed to Children (2011) recommendation for voluntary improvements in industry self-regulation of food marketing to children. As some of the most frequent advertisers to children, the cereal industry received considerable scrutiny in these reports. To their credit, cereal companies have implemented more improvements than most other food and beverage categories.

Encouragingly, parents' attitudes about cereals appear to be changing. A Rudd Center survey conducted annually since 2009 shows an increase in parents' perceptions that food marketing negatively affects their children's eating habits, including common cereal-company practices such as cartoon characters on packages, in-store promotions, advergames, and internet advertising (Harris, Fleming-Milici, Sarda, & Schwartz, 2012). The percent of parents who reported feeding their children sugared cereals daily declined significantly, from 27% in 2009 to 22% in 2013 (Harris, Fleming-Milici, & Liu, 2014). Notably, in 2013 and early 2014, Kellogg, General Mills, and Post reported declines in cereal sales that have affected their earnings (Cavale, 2014; Stock, 2013). News reports cite the cost of breakfast cereals and evolving consumer tastes in favor of healthier choices and on-the-go options, as well as parents' concerns about the high sugar content of cereals.

This case study in using scientific research to encourage industry actions to promote healthy food choices to children also demonstrates limitations of this approach. Notably, cereal companies have made only limited attempts to market low-sugar cereals to children, our primary request to them. Our meetings with the cereal companies revealed significant barriers to implementing such a major change in marketing strategy. Some appeared to remain convinced that high-sugar cereals are nutritious options for children. Others explained that dramatically altering their business model for children's cereals, which has been enormously successful for more than 30 years, would present an untenable business risk. This potential risk is exacerbated by legitimate concerns that a company choosing to 'do the right thing' would lose market share if all competitors did not make similar changes.

Findings also demonstrate the limits of industry self-regulation in producing meaningful change, even in the face of considerable public scrutiny of company practices. Only one company (Quaker, owned by PepsiCo) discontinued child-targeted marketing of high-sugar cereals. Perhaps this decision was easier because PepsiCo sold just one child-targeted cereal (*Cap'n Crunch*). Instead, the other cereal companies agreed to somewhat reduce the sugar content of their established children's cereal brands. General Mills and Kellogg appear to be exploring new market segments for some high-sugar cereals beyond young children.

Conversely, there is evidence that government regulation can lead to faster and more meaningful change. The threat of an investigation of Smart Choices by one state attorney general and the FDA prompted companies to quickly suspend its launch. In addition, although cereal companies may believe that marketing low-sugar cereals to children is impossible, it is notable that both Kellogg and General Mills have developed low-sugar versions of children's cereals (including *Froot Loops, Apple Jacks,* and *Cinnamon Toast Crunch*) to meet USDA's new nutrition guidelines for school meals (USDA, 2012). Apparently they believe that children will eat these cereals when served in schools, yet the reformulated versions are not generally available in supermarkets. However, the preferred approach to address unhealthy food marketing to children in most countries, as in the United States, has been to defer to industry self-regulation over government regulation or legislation (Hawkes, 2007).

Conclusion

In announcing the first *Cereal FACTS* report, Dr. Kelly Brownell, former Director of the Rudd Center stated, 'If there is to be any hope of protecting children from predatory marketing, either public outcry or government action will be necessary to force the companies to change'. As illustrated in this case study, further improvements in food marketing to children will require continued pressure from all directions. Big Food will likely continue promising to be part of the solution to childhood obesity and support parents' efforts to raise healthy children. Researchers must continue to independently evaluate the accuracy of companies' statements by examining the nutritional quality of products marketed to children and the extent and impact of child-directed marketing. Advocates must harness the research to mobilize parents and pressure companies to change. However, government policies that protect children from exposure to marketing of unhealthy products also may be necessary to ensure that food companies reform their food marketing practices to meaningfully contribute to improvements in children's diets.

Acknowledgement
We would like to thank the staff at the Rudd Center who contributed to the research outlined in this manuscript.

Funding
This research was supported by a grant from the Robert Wood Johnson Foundation.

References

Albertson, A. M., Affenito, S. G., Bauserman, R., Holschuh, N. M., Eldridge, A. L., & Barton, B. A. (2009). The relationship of ready-to-eat cereal consumption to nutrient intake, blood lipids, and body mass index of children as they age through adolescence. *Journal of the American Dietetic Association, 109*, 1557–1565.

Alvy, L. M., & Calvert, S. L. (2008). Food marketing on popular children's web sites: A content analysis. *Journal of the American Dietetic Association, 108*, 710–713.

Castetbon, K., Harris, J. L., & Schwartz, M. B. (2012). Purchases of ready-to-eat cereals vary across US household sociodemographic categories according to nutritional value and advertising targets. *Public Health Nutrition, 15*, 1456–1465.

Cavale, S. (2014, February 6). Kellogg revenue misses as cereal sales stay soggy. *Reuters.* Retrieved from http://www.reuters.com/article/2014/02/06/us-kellogg-results-idUSBREA150Y S20140206

Cho, S., Dietrich, M., Brown, C. J., Clark, C. A., & Block, G. (2003). The effect of breakfast type on total daily energy intake and body mass index: Results from the third national health and nutrition examination survey (NHANES III). *Journal of the American College of Nutrition, 22*, 296–302.

Clark, C., & Crockett, S. J. (2008). Concern over ready-to-eat breakfast cereals: Letter to the editor. *Journal of the American Dietetic Association, 108*, 1618–1619.

Federal Trade Commission. (2008). *Marketing food to children and adolescents. A review of industry expenditures, activities, and self-regulation.* A report to Congress. Retrieved from http://ftc.gov/os/2008/07/P064504foodmktingreport.pdf

Federal Trade Commission. (2012). A review of food marketing to children and adolescents: Follow-up report. Retrieved from http://www.ftc.gov/os/2012/12/121221foodmarketingreport.pdf

General Mills. (2014). Cereal. Part of the solution. Retrieved from http://cerealbenefits.com/home.html

Goren, A., Harris, J. L., Schwartz, M. B., & Brownell, K. D. (2010). Predicting support for restricting food marketing to youth. *Health Affairs, 29*, 419–424.

Harris, J. L., Fleming-Milici, F., & Liu, S. (2014). Survey of parents' attitudes about food marketing to children. [Unpublished data].

Harris, J. L., Fleming-Milici, F., Sarda, V., & Schwartz, M. B. (2012). *Food marketing to children and adolescents: What do parents think?* Rudd Center for Food Policy and Obesity, Yale University. Retrieved from http://www.yaleruddcenter.org/resources/upload/docs/what/reports/Rudd_Report_Parents_Survey_Food_Marketing_2012.pdf

Harris, J. L., Schwartz, M. B., & Brownell, K. D. (2010). Marketing foods to children and adolescents: Licensed characters and other promotions on packaged foods in the supermarket. *Public Health Nutrition, 13*, 409–417.

Harris, J. L., Schwartz, M. B., Brownell, K. D., Sarda, V., Dembek, C., Munsell, C., … Weinberg, M. (2012). *Cereal FACTS 2012: Limited progress in the nutrition quality and marketing of children's cereals.* Rudd Center for Food Policy and Obesity, Yale University. Retrieved from http://www.cerealfacts.org/media/Cereal_FACTS_Report_2012_7.12.pdf

Harris, J. L., Schwartz, M. B., Brownell, K. D., Sarda, V., Weinberg, M. E., Speers, S., … Byrnes-Enoch, H. (2009). *Cereal FACTS: Evaluating the nutrition quality and marketing of children's cereals.* Rudd Center for Food Policy and Obesity, Yale University. Retrieved from http://cerealfacts.org/media/Cereal_FACTS_Report_2009.pdf

Harris, J. L., Schwartz, M. B., Ustjanauskas, A., Ohri-Vachaspati, P., & Brownell, K. D. (2011). Effects of serving high-sugar cereals on children's breakfast-eating behavior. *Pediatrics, 127*, 71–76.

Harris, J. L., Speers, S. E., Schwartz, M. B., & Brownell, K. D. (2012). US food company branded advergames on the internet: Children's exposure and effects on snack consumption. *Journal of Children and Media, 6*, 51–68.

Harris, J. L., Thompson, J. M., Schwartz, M. B., & Brownell, K. D. (2011). Nutrition-related claims on children's cereals: What do they mean to parents and do they influence willingness to buy? *Public Health Nutrition, 14*, 2207–2212.

Harris, J. L., Weinberg, M. E., Javadizadeh, J., & Sarda, V. (2013). Monitoring food company marketing to children to spotlight best and worst practices. In J. D. Williams, K. E. Pasch, & C. A. Collins (Eds.), *Advances in communication research to reduce childhood obesity* (pp. 153–175). New York, NY: Springer Media.

Hawkes, C. (2007). Regulating and litigating in the public interest: Regulating food marketing to young people worldwide: Trends and policy drivers. *American Journal of Public Health, 97*, 1962–1973.

Institute of Medicine, Committee on Food Marketing and the Diets of Children and Youth. (2006). *Food marketing to children and youth: Threat or opportunity?* Washington, DC: National Academies Press.

Interagency Working Group on Food Marketed to Children. (2011). Preliminary proposed nutrition principles to guide industry self-regulatory efforts. Retrieved from http://www.ftc.gov/os/2011/04/110428foodmarketproposedguide.pdf

Johnson, R. K., Appel, L. J., Brands, M., Howard, B. V., Lefevre, M., Lustig, R. H., ... Wylie-Rosett, J. (2009). Dietary sugars intake and cardiovascular health. A scientific statement from the American Heart Association. *Journal of the American Heart Association, 120*, 1011–1020.

Kolish, E. D., & Enright, M. (2013). *The Children's Food & Beverage Advertising Initiative.* A report on compliance and progress during 2012. Retrieved from http://www.bbb.org/Global/Council_113/CFBAI%20Report%20on%20Compliance%20and%20Progress%20During%202012.pdf

Kunkel, D., McKinley, C., & Wright, P. (2009). *The impact of industry self-regulation on the nutritional quality of foods advertised on television to children.* Retrieved from www.children now.org/uploads/documents/adstudy_2009.pdf

LoDolce, M. E., Harris, J. L., & Schwartz, M. B. (2013). Sugar as part of a balanced breakfast? What cereal advertisements teach children about healthy eating. *Journal of Health Communication, 18*, 1293–1309.

NBC News. (2010). Post foods to cut some cereals' sugar content. Retrieved from http://www.nbc news.com/id/40796626/ns/health-diet_and_nutrition/t/post-foods-cut-some-cereals-sugar-con tent/#.Uz2BzxAVC5J

Neuman, W. (2009). For your health, Froot Loops. *The New York Times.* Retrieved from http://www.nytimes.com/2009/09/05/business/05smart.html?pagewanted=all&_r=0

Powell, L. M., Harris, J. L., & Fox, T. (2013). Food marketing expenditures aimed at youth: Putting the numbers in context. *American Journal of Preventive Medicine, 45*, 453–461.

Powell, L. M., Schermbeck, R. M., Szczpka, G., Chaloupka, F. J., & Braunschweig, C. L. (2011). Trends in the nutritional content of television food advertisements seen by children in the United States. *Archives of Pediatrics & Adolescent Medicine, 165*, 1078–1086.

Powell, L. M., Szczypka, G., & Chaloupka, F. J. (2007). Exposure to food advertising on television among US children. *Archives of Pediatrics & Adolescent Medicine, 161*, 553–560.

Ruiz, R. (2009). Smart choices fails. *Forbes.* Retrieved from http://www.forbes.com/2009/10/23/smart-choices-labeling-lifestyle-health-fda-food-labeling.html

Schwartz, M. B., Ross, C., Harris, J. L., Jernigan, D. H., Siegel, M., Ostroff, J., & Brownell, K. D. (2010). Breakfast cereal industry pledges to self-regulate advertising to youth: Will they improve the marketing landscape? *Journal of Public Health Policy, 31*, 59–73.

Schwartz, M. B., Vartanian, L., Wharton, C., & Brownell, K. D. (2008). Examining the nutritional quality of breakfast cereals marketed to children. *Journal of the American Dietetic Association, 108*, 702–705.

Skidmore, S. (2009, December 9). General Mills reducing sugar in kids' cereal, *USA Today.* Retrieved from http://usatoday30.usatoday.com/money/industries/food/2009-12-09-general-mills-cereals_N.htm

Smart Choices. (2009). Smart choices program postpones active operations. [Press release]. Retrieved from http://www.smartchoicesprogram.com/pr_091023_operations.html

Speers, S., Goren, A., Harris, J. L., Schwartz, M. B., & Brownell, K. D. (2009). *Public perceptions of food marketing to youth: Results of the Rudd Center Public Opinion Poll, May 2008.* Rudd Center for Food Policy and Obesity, Yale University. Retrieved from www.yaleruddcenter.org/resources/upload/docs/what/reports/RuddReportPublicPerceptionsFoodMarketingYouth2009.pdf

Stock, K. (2013). On-the-go Americans are ditching their cereal bowls. *Bloomberg Businessweek.* Retrieved from http://www.businessweek.com/articles/2013-08-02/on-the-go-americans-are-ditching-their-cereal-bowls

The White House. (2013). Remarks by the First Lady during White House convening on food marketing to children. [Press release]. Retrieved from http://www.whitehouse.gov/the-press-office/2013/09/18/remarks-first-lady-during-white-house-convening-food-marketing-children

Thompson, D., Franko, D. L., & Barton, B. A. (2008). Concern over ready-to-eat breakfast cereals. *Journal of the American Dietetic Association, 108*, 117–118.

US Department of Agriculture. (2010). My pyramid for kids. Retrieved April 4, 2014, from http://www.cnpp.usda.gov/MyPyramidforKids.htm

US Department of Agriculture. (2012). Nutrition standards for school meals. Retrieved April 21, 2014, from http://www.fns.usda.gov/cnd/Governance/Legislation/nutritionstandards.htm

Ustjanauskas, A., Eckman, B., Harris, J. L., Goren, A., Schwartz, M. B., & Brownell, K. D. (2010). *Focus groups with parents*. Rudd Center for Food Policy and Obesity, Yale University. Retrieved from http://www.yaleruddcenter.org/resources/upload/docs/what/reports/RuddReport_FocusGroupsParents_5.10.pdf

White House Task Force on Childhood Obesity. (2010). Solving the problem of childhood obesity within a generation. Retrieved from www.letsmove.gov/tfco_fullreport_may2010.pdf

Yale Rudd Center. (2014). Cereal FACTS in the news. Retrieved from http://cerealfacts.org/press.aspx

Big Soda's long shadow: news coverage of local proposals to tax sugar-sweetened beverages in Richmond, El Monte and Telluride

Laura Nixon, Pamela Mejia, Andrew Cheyne and Lori Dorfman

Berkeley Media Studies Group, Berkeley, CA, USA

In 2012 and 2013, Richmond and El Monte, CA, and Telluride, CO, became the first communities in the country to vote on citywide sugary drink taxes. In the face of massive spending from the soda industry, all three proposals failed at the ballot box, but the vigorous public debates they inspired provide valuable insights for future policy efforts. We analyzed local and national news coverage of the three proposals and found that pro-tax arguments appeared most frequently in the news. Advocates for the taxes focused primarily on the potential community health benefits the taxes could produce and the health harms caused by sodas. Tax opponents capitalized on the existing political tensions in each community, including racial and ethnic divisions in Richmond, anti-government attitudes in El Monte, and a culture of individualism in Telluride. Pro-tax arguments came mainly from city officials and public health advocates, while anti-tax forces recruited a wide range of people to speak against the tax. The soda industry itself was conspicuously absent from news coverage. Instead, in each community, the industry funded anti-tax coalition groups, whose affiliation with industry was often not acknowledged in the news. Our analysis of this coverage exposes how soda tax opponents used strategies established by the tobacco industry to fight regulation. Despite these defeats, tax advocates can take inspiration from more mature public health campaigns, which indicate that such policies may take many years to gain traction.

Introduction

Because of their association with a range of chronic diseases including type 2 diabetes, cardiovascular diseases, dental caries, and some cancers (Basen-Engquist & Chang, 2011; Flores, 2010; Vartanian, Schwartz, & Brownell, 2007), reducing the consumption of sugary drinks is a key public health objective. Sugary drinks are the largest source of added sugars in the American diet (Reedy & Krebs-Smith, 2010; Welsh, Sharma, Grellinger, & Vos, 2011), responsible for up to 43% of the increase in caloric intake over the past generation (Woodward-Lopez, Kao, & Ritchie, 2010). While soda consumption has declined over the last fifteen years (Kit, Fakhouri, Park, Nielsen, & Ogden, 2013), consumption of other sugary beverages such as sports and energy drinks has risen (Han & Powell, 2013).

Sugary beverages, and the marketing that promotes them, are also associated with substantial racial and ethnic health disparities. African-American and Latino communities, particularly children, have been strategically targeted by the sugary beverage industry (Grier & Kumanyika, 2008; Harris et al., 2011). They are exposed to significantly more advertising for sugary drinks (Harris et al., 2011; Kumanyika, Grier, Lancaster, & Lassiter, 2011) and purchase significantly more sweetened beverages than their white counterparts (Piernas, Ng, & Popkin, 2013). Among adults, energy intake from sugary drink consumption is higher among Latinos and African-Americans than non-Hispanic whites (Ogden, Kit, Carroll, & Park, 2011).

Due in part to the success of excise taxes on tobacco products in reducing consumption, taxing sugar-sweetened beverages has been identified as a key policy lever to reduce consumption of sugary drinks and to fund nutrition and physical activity programs (Andreyeva, Chaloupka, & Brownell, 2011; Andreyeva, Long, & Brownell, 2010; Brownell & Frieden, 2009; Brownell et al., 2009; Chaloupka & Davidson, 2010; Chaloupka, Powell, & Chriqui, 2011; Powell, Chriqui, Khan, Wada, & Chaloupka, 2013). Young people are likely to be especially responsive to taxes on sugary drinks due to their limited resources (Andreyeva et al., 2011). Soda taxes also have the potential to improve public health by generating revenue for programs to prevent obesity and disease or to fund health care services to manage illnesses linked to sugary drink consumption (Brownell & Frieden, 2009; Wang, Coxson, Shen, Goldman, & Bibbins-Domingo, 2012).

However, lessons from tobacco control suggest that the beverage industry will strongly oppose taxes on their products, including by mounting extensive public relations campaigns to convince voters that measures to restrict their products or marketing practices are unnecessary (Brownell & Frieden, 2009; Brownell et al., 2010; Pomeranz, 2014). Indeed, led by the American Beverage Association trade group, the non-alcoholic beverage industry has spent tens of millions of dollars defeating the more than two dozen municipal and state soda taxes proposed around the country since 2009 (California Center for Public Health Advocacy, 2011; Grynbaum, 2012; Zingale, 2012). Nevertheless, public health advocates are continuing their attempts to reduce sugary drink consumption through taxation (American Heart Association, 2013; Friedman & Brownell, 2012), with new tax proposals unveiled and others under consideration (Knobel, 2014; Miller, 2013; Ottier, 2014; Wilkey, 2013).

The soda tax measures in Richmond and El Monte, CA, and Telluride, CO, were the first to be placed on a municipal ballot and decided by voters. Each proposed a 1-cent-per-ounce levy on sugary beverages by volume, but the three cities designated the potential revenue from the taxes quite differently. In California, Proposition 13, a voter-approved law passed in the late 1970s, stipulates that for a local jurisdiction like a city or county to pass a new tax, any earmarked tax must receive two-thirds of the electoral vote, compared to just 50% of the vote if the revenue is directed to the general fund. In Richmond and El Monte, revenues from the taxes were directed to the general fund, which meant that the taxes required only a simple majority to pass. However, tax supporters also proposed non-binding companion measures recommending that the respective city governments spend the revenue on specific purposes. In Richmond, a 'majority minority' city with a disproportionately low-income population (US Census, 2010), the revenues were to be dedicated to physical activity and other obesity prevention programs (Smart Voter, 2012). In El Monte, a predominantly Latino city (US Census, 2010) facing bankruptcy, officials intended to use the tax primarily to fund vital city services, though Mayor Andre Quintero acknowledged the importance of the tax to support health programs as well (Pamer & Lopez, 2012). In Telluride, a relatively affluent ski destination of some 2300 residents (US Census, 2010), the measure dedicated funds to youth-focused physical activity programs nearing the end of their federal grant funding. Although the funds were earmarked, in Colorado, this tax required only a simple majority.

The failed proposals generated substantial news, opinion, and industry trade press coverage. Analyzing such news coverage matters because in a democratic society, the news helps set the agenda for public policy debates (Dearing & Rogers, 1996; Scheufele & Tewksbury, 2007). Journalists' decisions about whether and how to cover an issue can raise its profile, while issues that are not covered by the news are less visible and often remain outside public discourse and policy debate (McCombs & Reynolds, 2009). New media platforms are changing the way people access news, but newspapers (including their online versions) continue to influence local and national policy debate. The majority of newspaper readers are registered voters, and traditional news outlets remain a key source of information for the majority of news consumers (Newspaper Association of America, 2012; Sasseen, Olmstead, & Mitchell, 2013).

Previous analyses of soda tax debates found that pro-soda tax arguments were more common in the news than anti-tax arguments, that key pro-tax messages include the health and financial benefits of taxation, and that concerns about financial harm and the proper role of government are central anti-tax messages (Jou, Niederdeppe, Barry, & Gollust, 2014; Niederdeppe, Gollust, Jarlenski, Nathanson, & Barry, 2013). Past research has also examined the beverage industry's strategies to fight regulation (Brownell & Warner, 2009), which include creating and funding community-based front groups to speak for them (Yanamadala, Bragg, Roberto, & Brownell, 2012).

This paper assesses the news coverage of the first three municipal soda tax initiatives to be decided by voters. Given the potential for beverage taxes to support public health, we wanted to understand the frequency and type of pro- and anti-tax arguments to which the voting public has been exposed.

Methods

We conducted an ethnographic content analysis of news reports on soda tax initiatives in Richmond, El Monte, and Telluride. Ethnographic content analysis is a reflexive method in which researchers develop initial categories and 'variables,' but others are allowed and expected to emerge throughout the study (Altheide, 1987).

Sample selection

For Richmond and El Monte, we searched the *Nexis* news database for 'All English Language News' published between November 2011 and January 2013 that mentioned at least one of the tax proposals. We supplemented this search with reviews of the online archives of English- and Spanish-language news sources not included in the *Nexis* database that we identified as important outlets covering these campaigns from our ongoing media monitoring of soda policy and marketing issues (Berkeley Media Studies Group, 2014), including the online and print archives of industry trade press publications such as *Beverage Digest*. We eliminated duplicate and irrelevant articles, e.g. articles about tax policies in Richmond, Virginia. Because of the large number of English-language news articles, we randomly selected for our sample every other relevant article from the *Nexis* and news outlet queries. Since we identified only a small number of Spanish-language and industry press news pieces, we included all of these in our analysis.

For Telluride, we used a comparable set of search terms to query the *Nexis* database for articles published between November 2012 and January 2014 that mentioned the Telluride tax proposal. We supplemented this with articles from the online and print archives of industry trade press publications, a Google News search, and the online archives of *The Telluride Daily Planet* and *The Watch*, two local news sources not included in the *Nexis* database. As there were comparatively few articles about the Telluride proposal, we included all of them in our final sample. A list of search terms and sources for all campaigns is included in Appendix 1 (see web appendix).

Coding

We designed our coding protocol by first incorporating arguments for and against soda taxes identified from our prior studies (Mejia, Nixon, Cheyne, Dorfman, & Quintero, 2014) and ongoing monitoring of news coverage of soda regulation policy debates. For each argument, coders recorded the speaker and identified the community to which the speaker referred. We revised this protocol using an iterative process (Altheide, 1987) to adjust the instrument until we reached acceptable intercoder agreement adjusting for chance using Krippendorff's alpha ($\alpha > .72$) (Krippendorff, 2009).

Results

What kind of news did soda taxes create, and when?

Our final sample included 378 relevant articles about the three tax proposals. We analyzed 222 articles that focused primarily on Richmond, 103 that focused on Telluride, and 53 about El Monte. Articles about each proposal most often appeared in the weeks immediately before and after the elections during which they were decided or when the proposal was first placed on that city's ballot (Figure 1).

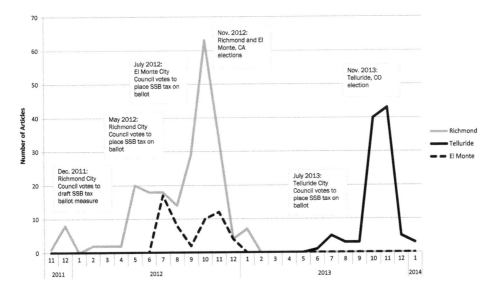

Figure 1. Newspaper articles about soda tax proposals in Richmond and El Monte, CA and Telluride, CO, 2011–2014 ($n = 378$).

Across the communities, the majority of the coverage consisted of straight news stories (55%). The remaining 45% was opinion articles, including letters to the editor (32%), op-eds (17%), blogs (16%), and editorials (9%). Within each community, however, the proportion of news and opinion coverage varied widely. In Richmond, 40% of coverage was opinion pieces, just over half of which favoured the soda tax. Opinion pieces dominated news in Telluride (67% of articles), but in El Monte they comprised just 26% of soda tax coverage. In both communities, the majority of opinion pieces opposed soda taxes (58 and 80%, respectively). All of the unsigned editorials written about the issue took an anti-tax position.

Framing the soda tax debates: Who said what in Richmond, Telluride, and El Monte?

We found 3013 instances of arguments for or against the taxes in coverage about the three soda tax proposals. The most frequent speakers from all three communities were city officials (such as Richmond City Councilmember Jeff Ritterman and El Monte Mayor Andre Quintero), community residents, public health advocates (such as Harold Goldstein of the California Center for Public Health Advocacy), and representatives from the local business community (Table 1; Figures 2(a)–2(d) [see web appendix]). Fewer distinct voices appeared in the news to support soda taxes, primarily city officials and public health advocates, while a broader range of stakeholders, including local business owners, community residents, city officials, leaders of local community groups, medical professionals, and religious leaders spoke against the taxes. Many of these anti-tax speakers were funded by the local anti-tax groups set up by the soda industry, but this affiliation was often not made explicit in news coverage. On the other hand, speakers who were explicitly identified as soda industry representatives appeared infrequently in the news. When they did it was speakers representing industry trade groups, not company officials, who ridiculed efforts to reduce obesity by addressing sugary drinks, as in this rhetorical question from the American Beverage Association: 'What part of

Table 1. Prevalence of speakers quoted in soda tax debates by community (n = 2754).

Speaker	Richmond (% of total)	Telluride (% of total)	El Monte (% of total)
City official	36	12	25
Community resident	18	28	13
Public health advocate	7	13	4
Business community	5	12	7
Kick the Can	0	17	0
Medical personnel/researcher	8	2	4
Opinion author	5	4	13
Local anti-tax coalition	6	2	2
Soda industry representative	2	3	3
General 'opponents'	4	2	5
General 'supporters'	3	2	5
African-American organization	3	0	0
Religious leader	2	0	0

Notes: Table 1 includes a subset of the arguments that appeared in the news. It does not include statements that were part of the articles but were not linked to a specific speaker (n = 259), such as unattributed statements about the prevalence of obesity.

"full calorie soda sales have declined 12.5 percent over the past decade while obesity rates have increased" don't you understand?' (American Beverage Association, 2012).

Pro-tax arguments across all three communities focused on the health benefits of the tax and the health harms caused by sugary drinks (Table 2). There was substantially more variation in the arguments used by tax opponents, who employed a range of anti-tax arguments based on the character and concerns of each community.

Richmond

Advocates in Richmond, where the soda tax was proposed as a public health measure, emphasized the community-wide health benefits they expected from the tax. Richmond council member Jeff Ritterman, the author of the proposal and a retired cardiologist, was among the most enthusiastic proponents of the health argument, saying the tax would create 'a healthier future for our children' (Smith & Ritterman, 2012). Other supporters specifically pointed out the benefits to the community from the health promotion programs the tax would fund. Richmond resident Jonathan Perez, for example, was reported as saying 'it's worth paying a few cents to have more sports fields and recreational activities' (Pulido, 2012). Public health advocate Harold Goldstein was quoted critiquing the soda industry's flurry of activities to undermine the campaign, contrasting how residents are 'using the power of democracy to say we want to change this [health harms from sugary drinks] ... but the beverage industry is using the enormous power of its pocketbook to try and crush it' (Lee, 2012).

Richmond's history of racial animosity was apparent in news about the soda tax proposal. Tax opponents representing the African-American community in Richmond, many of them part of the industry-funded Community Coalition Against Beverage Taxes (CCABT), argued that the tax was racist or regressive, characterizing it as a 'racist ploy' (Whitney, 2012) and a way to 'marginalize people of color' (Kenyon, 2011). Nat Bates, a veteran city council member, accused the mostly white Richmond City Council members who proposed the tax of 'using the black community to pass a measure for us without consulting us' (Onshi, 2012). Some news coverage suggested political motives behind claims of racism present in the campaign. Describing the process by which the beverage industry aligned itself with the Latino and African-American communities in Richmond, reporter Wendi Jonassen wrote, 'BMWL & Partners [the PR firm that represented the industry] was well aware of the racial divide within the city, and deftly exploited it' (Jonassen, 2013).

Industry opponents also used the two-step process of sending tax revenues into the general fund and then designating proceeds to obesity prevention programs to sow doubt about the purpose of the tax and raise questions about the motives of pro-tax advocates. Public relations executive and CCABT spokesperson Chuck Finnie, for example, insinuated in the news that advocates were lying to residents. 'Not a single penny will go to anti-obesity programs, but the proponents are misrepresenting it to say it will' (Rogers, 2012).

Telluride

The most common pro-tax argument in Telluride centered on the potential of the proposed tax to improve the health of the community. Proponents made the case for the tax to support health by emphasizing that it would fund the Physical Education Program as a means to 'keep [local] kids moving' (Hughes, 2013). One local mother described

Table 2. Prevalence of key pro- and anti-soda tax arguments during news coverage of three recent policy debates ($n = 3013$).

Argument	Core position	Core issue	Richmond (% total)	Telluride (% total)	El Monte (% total)
Pro-tax arguments					
Tax will improve community health	The tax will improve health by reducing consumption of harmful products and increasing funding for obesity prevention	The issue is whether soda taxes improve community health	16	16	13
Soda harms health	Sodas are implicated in obesity and are uniquely harmful to people's health	The issue is whether sodas harm public health	14	12	9
Big Soda undermines democracy	The soda industry is spending excessively on its anti-tax campaign and behaves dishonestly in its marketing	The issue is the appropriateness of the beverage industry's actions	12	9	13
Obesity is a pressing problem	Obesity is a public health problem that warrants action	The issue is whether obesity presents a threat to public health	10	9	8
Ripple effect	The tax will set a precedent for other communities	The issue is how the tax will affect future policy actions	4	4	0
Innovative and worthwhile policy	The soda tax is an innovative policy that will benefit the community	The issue is whether the policy is appropriate	2	4	2
Business as usual	Local businesses will be able to implement the tax without harmful economic consequences	The issue is how the tax will impact the community's economic health	2	3	1
Economic boon	The tax will provide much-needed tax revenues for city services and infrastructure	The issue is how the tax will impact the community's economic health	0	0	17
Low-income communities of color benefit	The tax will have the greatest positive effect on low-income communities of color	The issue is how the tax will affect low-income communities of color	1	<1	0
Anti-tax arguments					
Economic harm	The tax will cost local businesses money, raise prices, and harm community residents	The issue is how the tax will impact the community's economic health	11	13	18

(Continued)

Table 2. (Continued).

Argument	Core position	Core issue	Richmond (% total)	Telluride (% total)	El Monte (% total)
Ineffective solution	Soda taxes are an ineffective solution to a serious problem	The issue is whether soda taxes improve community health	9	12	6
Government intrusion	Government is restricting residents' right to make their own choices	The issue is whether government action is appropriate	3	8	10
Racist and regressive	This is a paternalistic, regressive tax that will harm low-income communities of color	The issue is how the tax will affect low-income communities of color	6	1	0
A blank check to city hall	The tax will not improve health because the revenue will not support obesity prevention programs	The issue is whether proceeds from the tax will fund obesity prevention	3	<1	3
Don't blame soda	Soda is unfairly targeted. Obesity results from many factors, not just drinking soda	The issue is whether sodas harm public health	3	1	0
Soda industry defends the community	The soda industry has the community's best interest at heart	The issue is the appropriateness of the beverage industry's actions	1	2	0
Obesity is not a priority	The community has higher-priority problems	The issue is whether obesity presents a true threat to public health	<1	3	0
Both sides receive funding	Soda tax supporters and opponents are bringing in outside money to tell the local community what to do	The issue is whether soda tax advocates have behaved appropriately during the campaign	0	2	0

Source: Adapted from Ryan (1991).

in glowing terms her daughter's experience, concluding, 'I am prepared to pay an extra 12 cents for my occasional soda … if it means the continuation of these programs for the children of Telluride' (Huff, 2013). Spokespeople also explained the health harms the tax would address, as voiced by local advocates Emo Overall and Bridget Taddonio: 'We have an obesity epidemic in our nation and we now know that sugary drinks are the biggest single contributor' (Overall & Taddonio, 2013). The local pro-tax Kick the Can coalition – the leading proponent quoted in Telluride coverage – also connected arguments about community well-being to the role of the soda industry and its allies in undermining health, urging residents to 'take on big business to do something wonderful for the health of our community and it's[sic] children' (Taddonio, 2013).

As in Richmond, anti-tax arguments were tailored to the character and concerns of the town. For example, Telluride tax opponents questioned if residents of their 'athletically oriented ski town' (Roisman, 2013a) were truly at risk for obesity and consequently, whether a tax to support obesity prevention programs was necessary, since 'Telluride children are a lot healthier than most' (Adams, 2013). One long-term resident observed, '[I've] looked at children in the schoolyard and on the streets of Telluride and, for the life of me, I don't see obesity as a local problem' (Roisman, 2013a).

Telluride residents took pride not only in their children's health and athleticism, but also in their town's reputation as a fiercely independent 'Civil Liberties Safe Zone' (Lundeen, 2013) where 'everyone does their own thing' (Lynch, 2013). Some tax opponents tapped into this civic pride to raise opposition to the specter of 'manipulation from outside interests' (Roisman, 2013b). The soda tax effort in Telluride was a local campaign, but because they had the support of public health advocates from around the country such as the California Center for Public Health Advocacy, opponents characterized soda tax advocates as 'outsiders blowing into town' who were 'determined to tell Telluride what to do when it comes to our health' (Harnish, 2013). Bob Harnish, head of the industry-funded anti-tax group 'No on 2A,' called into question the legitimacy of local soda tax advocates when he characterized their proposal as 'bothersome, because it's portrayed as a local measure, but it's actually coming from the California Center for Public Health Advocacy' (Klingsporn, 2013). The divisions between Telluride residents and outsiders were emphasized by arguments that chastised local tax supporters for receiving out-of-state-funding (Roisman, 2013b).

El Monte

The most common pro-tax argument in El Monte focused on the economic impact the tax would have on the city. Supporters were reported as saying that a sugary drink tax would balance the city budget and '[address] long-term structural budget deficits' (Velazquez, 2012b). Even when supporters touted health benefits, their comments in the news emphasized that the tax was first about raising revenue for the general fund, as when Mayor Andre Quintero said, '[T]here are significant financial hurdles that we need to start dealing with now, so having this type of tax as an option brings in revenue and hopefully encourages individuals to make healthier choices' (Velazquez, 2012a). As in Richmond, proponents also criticized the soda industry's activities; the El Monte ballot language even suggested that soda companies 'want to avoid paying their fair share and don't care about the safety and health of El Monte's neighborhoods' (Velazquez, 2012c).

Anti-tax arguments in El Monte also highlighted economic implications, with reports of local business owners lamenting that their customers 'don't want to pay higher prices, and in this economy, fewer of them can actually afford to' (Ballesteros-Coronel, 2012). Other detractors framed the tax as an example of government overreach and mismanagement, taking advantage of the fact that the city was facing the prospect of bankruptcy. Former City Councilman Art Barrios, for example, was quoted claiming that El Monte politicians were 'trying to make up for years of overspending by taxing beverages like sports drinks, ice teas, bubble teas, horchata and agua fresca' (Velazquez, 2012c). Barrios' statement echoed the beverage industry's multi-lingual anti-tax campaign in El Monte; the industry targeted different groups with claims that the tax would impact beverages that are culturally relevant to specific ethnic communities, such as horchata and bubble tea (Jou et al., 2014).

Discussion

The efforts to tax sugary drinks in Richmond, El Monte, and Telluride produced vigorous and at times rancorous debate in the news between supporters and opponents. Overall, pro-tax arguments appeared more frequently in the news, consistent with previous analyses (Niederdeppe et al., 2013). Tax supporters' arguments emphasized the taxes as an effective response to a public health crisis. Opposition arguments varied based on the context in each community. Tax opponents capitalized on racial divisions in diverse, working-class Richmond, while in the outdoorsy ski town of Telluride, they argued that obesity was not a pressing problem and worried about government intrusion. In El Monte, detractors predicted the tax would bring financial ruin.

Support for the tax in these communities came from a relatively small set of impassioned advocates, while a wider range of speakers, from local business owners to clergy, voiced opposition. The soda industry was conspicuously absent from the news, but many of those who spoke against the tax were part of local, industry-funded anti-tax coalitions, despite not being identified as such, even when they were receiving direct payments from the beverage industry. This may be a fairly recent development: an earlier analysis of soda taxes in the news found that anti-tax arguments were mostly voiced by beverage industry groups and pro-industry coalitions (Niederdeppe et al., 2013).

Implications

Like earlier analyses, our investigation of the news found that although the soda tax proposals in our study ultimately failed, the newspaper coverage about them was mostly positive (Niederdeppe et al., 2013). One potential reason for the fact that the taxes failed in spite of positive news coverage is that the news was just one influence on voters, and the soda industry poured millions of dollars into paid advertising, phone banking, door-to-door canvassing, and other efforts (Allen, 2012; Drange, 2012). In addition, while pro-tax arguments in the news mainly came from a few politicians and public health advocates, anti-tax forces recruited a wide range of local stakeholders to speak in the news, and these spokespeople, and the arguments they made, may have been more successful at convincing voters. Advocates for similar policies might want to pay particular attention to cultivating a range of spokespeople and exploring which spokespeople are most effective in these debates.

In each of the communities we studied, how the tax proposals were received reflected the existing community context, including racial divisions in Richmond, anti-government sentiment in El Monte, and a strong culture of individualism in Telluride.

The industry's approach mirrored the strategies employed by other industries such as Big Tobacco to affect news coverage and undermine campaigns to advance public health policies (Brownell, 2012; Brownell & Warner, 2009; Dorfman, Cheyne, Friedman, Wadud, & Gottlieb, 2012; Glantz & Balbach, 2000; Menashe, 1998; Proctor, 2006, 2011; Swisher & Reese, 1992; Yach & Bialous, 2001). Much like tobacco companies, the soda industry formed local community coalitions who spoke for them in the news (Apollonio & Bero, 2007a, 2007b; Brownell & Warner, 2009; Samuels & Glantz, 1991; Yanamadala et al., 2012). Unlike in earlier analyses of soda tax campaigns, however, we found that the soda industry itself was largely absent from news coverage of the soda taxes. In the future, public health advocates and researchers could explore whether pointing out the soda industry's stealth campaign tactics, or its marketing practices that prioritize self-interested profits over community health, are helpful in building support for soda taxes.

Like other industries facing policies that aim to address the health harms caused by their products and corporate practices, the soda industry has spent millions to defeat every tax measure proposed to date. In Richmond, for example, they spent almost as much as the tax would have raised in a year (Oatman, 2012). During these campaigns, however, public health advocates have successfully generated news coverage – sometimes more than their opponents – about the health harms of sugary drinks and policy options to address them. Informed by the lessons from more mature public health efforts such as tobacco, public health advocates can take comfort in the fact that enacting public health policies and making meaningful changes to our environment takes time. In tobacco control, advocates worked on clean indoor air policies for years before Duluth, MN, passed one of the first in 2000 – and then over the next 14 years, 39 states strengthened their policies (Centers for Disease Control and Prevention, 2014). Although the campaign to tax sugary drinks is still young, there is early evidence that even when soda tax proposals are unsuccessful, they increase awareness about the health harms of soda and potentially reduce consumption (Ravdin, 2014). In this view, which deserves further investigation, even failed campaigns can act as public health education tools, laying the groundwork for future public health victories.

Conflict of interest

We certify that there is no conflict of interest with any financial organization regarding the material discussed in the manuscript.

Funding

This paper was commissioned by the Robert Wood Johnson Foundation through its Healthy Eating Research program. The research which contributed to this analysis was supported in part by the California Endowment, and by the Robert Wood Johnson Foundation through its Healthy Eating Research Foundation [Grant Numbers CAS012, CAS016].

References

Adams, S. (2013, October 16). Sugary beverage tax strikes a nerve. *The Watch*.
Allen, S. (2012, October 29). Ad blitz aims to drown soda tax: El Monte mayor saw measure as a slam dunk. Then the drink makers declared war. *Los Angeles Times*.

Altheide, D. L. (1987). Reflections: ethnographic content analysis. *Qualitative Sociology, 10,* 65–77. doi:10.1007/bf00988269

American Beverage Association. (2012, September 18). A tale of two politicians. *Sip and Savor Blog.*

American Heart Association. (2013). *Decreasing sugar-sweetened beverage consumption: Policy approaches to address obesity.* Retrieved March 14, 2014, from http://www.heart.org/idc/groups/heart-public/@wcm/@adv/documents/downloadable/ucm_453908.pdf

Andreyeva, T., Chaloupka, F. J., & Brownell, K. D. (2011). Estimating the potential of taxes on sugar-sweetened beverages to reduce consumption and generate revenue. *Preventive Medicine, 52,* 413–416. doi: http://dx.doi.org/10.1016/j.ypmed.2011.03.013

Andreyeva, T, Long, M. W., & Brownell, K. D. (2010). The impact of food prices on consumption: A systematic review of research on the price elasticity of demand for food. *American Journal of Public Health, 100,* 216–222.

Apollonio, D. E., & Bero, L. A. (2007a). Industry front groups: A tobacco case study. *Journal of Consumer Protection and Food Safety, 2,* 341–348.

Apollonio, D. E., & Bero, L. A. (2007b). The creation of industry front groups: The tobacco industry and "get government off our back". *American Journal of Public Health, 97,* 419–427.

Ballesteros-Coronel, M. (2012, October 10). Empresarios de El Monte se oponen a Medida H. [El Monte businesspeople oppose Measure H]. *El Mensajero.*

Basen-Engquist, K., & Chang, M. (2011). Obesity and cancer risk: Recent review and evidence. *Current Oncology Reports, 13,* 71–76.

Berkeley Media Studies Group. (2014). *Building capacity to make the case for healthier beverage environments.* Retrieved November 25, 2014, from http://www.bmsg.org/about/projects/building-capacity-to-make-the-case-for-healthier-beverage-environments

Brownell, K. D. (2012). Thinking forward: The quicksand of appeasing the food industry. *PLoS Medicine, 9*(7), doi:10.1371/journal.pmed.1001254

Brownell, K. D., Farley, T., Willett, W. C., Popkin, B. M., Chaloupka, F. J., Thompson, J. W., & Ludwig, D. S. (2009). The public health and economic benefits of taxing sugar-sweetened beverages. *New England Journal of Medicine, 361,* 1599–1605. doi:10.1056/NEJMhpr0905723

Brownell, K. D., & Frieden, T. R. (2009). Ounces of prevention – The public policy case for taxes on sugared beverages. *New England Journal of Medicine, 360,* 1805–1808. doi:10.1056/NEJMp0902392

Brownell, K. D., Kersh, R., Ludwig, D. S., Post, R. C., Puhl, R. M., Schwartz, M. B., & Willett, W. C. (2010). Personal responsibility and obesity: A constructive approach to a controversial issue. *Health Affairs, 29,* 379–387. doi:10.1377/hlthaff.2009.0739

Brownell, K. D., & Warner, K. E. (2009). The perils of ignoring history: Big tobacco played dirty and millions died. How similar is big food? *Milbank Quarterly, 87,* 259–294.

California Center for Public Health Advocacy. (2011). *Soda industry ups political spending to fight proposed sugary drink taxes.* Retrieved April 30, 2014, from http://www.kickthecan.info/soda-industry-political-spending

Centers for Disease Control and Prevention. (2014). *State tobacco activities tracking and evaluation (STATE) system.* Retrieved April 14, 2014, from http://www.cdc.gov/tobacco/statesystem

Chaloupka, F. J., & Davidson, P. A. (2010). *Applying tobacco control lessons to obesity: Taxes and other pricing strategies to reduce consumption.* Retrieved from http://publichealthlawcenter.org/sites/default/files/resources/tclc-syn-obesity-2010.pdf

Chaloupka, F. J., Powell, L. M., & Chriqui, J. F. (2011). Sugar-sweetened beverage taxation as public health policy-lessons from tobacco. *Choices, 26*(3).

Dearing, J. W., & Rogers, E. M. (1996). *Agenda-setting.* Thousand Oaks, CA: Sage.

Dorfman, L., Cheyne, A., Friedman, L. C., Wadud, A., & Gottlieb, M. (2012). Soda and tobacco industry corporate social responsibility campaigns: How do they compare? *PLoS Medicine, 9*(6).

Drange, M. (2012, November 2). Soda industry pours millions into campaign to defeat Richmond soda tax. *The Bay Citizen.*

Flores, G. (2010). Racial and ethnic disparities in the health and health care of children. *Pediatrics, 125*, e979–e1020.

Friedman, R., & Brownell, K. D. (2012). *Sugar-sweetened beverage taxes: An updated policy brief.* Yale Rudd Center. Retrieved March 14, 2014, from http://www.yaleruddcenter.org/resources/upload/docs/what/reports/Rudd_Policy_Brief_Sugar_Sweetened_Beverage_Taxes.pdf

Glantz, S. A., & Balbach, E. D. (2000). *Tobacco war: Inside the California battles.* Berkeley, CA: University of California Press.

Grier, S. A., & Kumanyika, S. K. (2008). The context for choice: Health implications of targeted food and beverage marketing to African Americans. *American Journal of Public Health, 98*, 1616–1629. doi:10.2105/ajph.2007.115626

Grynbaum, M. M. (2012, July 1). Soda makers begin their push against New York ban. *New York Times.*

Han, E., & Powell, L. M. (2013). Consumption patterns of sugar-sweetened beverages in the United States. *Journal of the Academy of Nutrition and Dietetics, 113*, 43–53. doi: http://dx.doi.org/10.1016/j.jand.2012.09.016

Harnish, B. (2013, October 11). Stranger in town: The sugar tax. *Telluride Daily Planet.*

Harris, J. L., Schwartz, M. B., Brownell, K. D., Javadizadeh, J., Weinberg, M., Sarda, V., … Mejia, P. (2011). *Sugary drink FACTS: Evaluating sugary drink nutrition and marketing to youth.* New Haven, CT. Retrieved from http://www.sugarydrinkfacts.org/resources/SugaryDrinkFACTS_Report.pdf

Huff, B. (2013, October 20). Telluride mom for 2A. *Telluride Daily Planet.*

Hughes, M. (2013, October 30). Yes on 2A. *Telluride Daily Planet.*

Jonassen, W. (2013, January 23). Race-baiting in Richmond. *East Bay Express.*

Jou, J., Niederdeppe, J., Barry, C. L., & Gollust, S. E. (2014). Strategic messaging to promote taxation of sugar-sweetened beverages: Lessons from recent political campaigns. *American Journal of Public Health, 104*, 847–853. doi:10.2105/ajph.2013.301679

Kenyon, A. (2011, December 13). Richmond moves forward with Soda Tax. *The Bay Citizen.*

Kit, B. K., Fakhouri, T. H. I., Park, S., Nielsen, S. J., & Ogden, C. L. (2013). Trends in sugar-sweetened beverage consumption among youth and adults in the United States: 1999–2010. *American Journal of Clinical Nutrition, 98*, 180–188. doi:10.3945/ajcn.112.057943

Klingsporn, K. (2013, October 13). Sugar, obesity and the role of government. *Telluride Daily Planet.*

Knobel, L. (2014, February 12). Will Berkeley be first in nation to impose soda tax? *BerkeleySide.*

Krippendorff, K. (2009). *The content analysis reader.* Thousand Oaks, CA: Sage.

Kumanyika, S., Grier, S. A., Lancaster, K., & Lassiter, V. (2011). *Impact of sugar-sweetened beverage consumption on Black Americans' health.* Retrieved November 25, 2014, from http://www.aacorn.org/uploads/files/AACORNSSBBrief2011.pdf

Lee, C. (2012, November 4). Study: Soda tax would boost health of Latinos, blacks. *The Bay Citizen.*

Lundeen, P. (2013, June 30). Education, not taxes. *Telluride Daily Planet.*

Lynch, D. (2013, October 20). The Telluride beverage tax isn't the answer. *Telluride Daily Planet.*

McCombs, M., & Reynolds, A. (2009). How the news shapes our civic agenda. In J. Bryant & M. B. Oliver (Eds.), *Media effects: Advances in theory and research* (pp. 1–17). New York, NY: Taylor & Francis.

Mejia, P., Nixon, L., Cheyne, A., Dorfman, L., & Quintero, F. (2014). *Issue 21: Two communities, two debates: News coverage of soda tax proposals in Richmond and El Monte.* Berkeley, CA. Retrieved August 28, 2014, from http://www.bmsg.org/sites/default/files/bmsg_issue21_sodataxnews.pdf

Menashe, C. L. (1998). The power of a frame: An analysis of newspaper coverage of tobacco issues-United States, 1985-1996. *Journal of Health Communication, 3*, 307–325. doi:10.1080/108107398127139.

Miller, E. (2013, February 7). Soda tax discussed by lawmakers. *Hawaii Tribune Herald.*

Newspaper Association of America. (2012, February 15). Newspaper readers vote, and voters read newspapers.

Niederdeppe, J., Gollust, S. E., Jarlenski, M. P., Nathanson, A. M., & Barry, C. L. (2013). News coverage of sugar-sweetened beverage taxes: Pro- and antitax arguments in public discourse. *American Journal of Public Health, 103*, e92–e98. doi:10.2105/AJPH.2012.301023

Oatman, M. (2012, November 7). The Soda Tax Lost. Now What? *Mother Jones.*

Ogden, C. L., Kit, B. K., Carroll, M. D., & Park, S. (2011). *NCHS data brief: Consumption of sugar drinks in the United States, 2005–2008.* Centers for Disease Control and Prevention. Retrieved March 14, 2014, from http://www.cdc.gov/nchs/data/databriefs/db71.htm

Onshi, N. (2012). California city savors role in fighting "Big Soda". *New York Times.*

Ottier, M. (2014, February 18). Illinois "soda tax" proposal. *KWQC Local News.*

Overall, E. M., & Taddonio, B. (2013, July 31). The sugary drink tax explained. *Telluride Daily Planet.*

Pamer, M., & Lopez, L. (2012, July 24). El Monte declares fiscal emergency, can put soda tax on November ballot. *NBC 4: Southern California.*

Piernas, C., Ng, S. W., & Popkin, B. (2013). Trends in purchases and intake of foods and beverages containing caloric and low-calorie sweeteners over the last decade in the United States. *Pediatric Obesity, 8*, 294–306. doi:10.1111/j.2047-6310.2013.00153.x

Pomeranz, J. L. (2014). Sugary beverage tax policy: Lessons learned from tobacco. *American Journal of Public Health, 104*, e13–e15. doi:10.2105/ajph.2013.301800

Powell, L. M., Chriqui, J. F., Khan, T., Wada, R., & Chaloupka, F. J. (2013). Assessing the potential effectiveness of food and beverage taxes and subsidies for improving public health: A systematic review of prices, demand and body weight outcomes. *Obesity Reviews, 14*, 110–128. doi:10.1111/obr.12002.

Proctor, R. N. (2006). "Everyone knew but no one had proof": Tobacco industry use of medical history expertise in US courts, 1990–2002. *Tobacco Control, 15*, iv117–iv25.

Proctor, R. N. (2011). *Golden holocaust: Origins of the cigarette catastrophe and the case for abolition.* Berkeley, CA: University of California Press.

Pulido, T. (2012, November 7). Soda tax lost, but Richmond still won (sort of). *Richmond Pulse.*

Ravdin, G. (2014). Sugar sweetened beverage polling report. In *Using the right messages for sugar sweetened beverages: Results from research in Los Angeles, California and Vermont.* Webinar. Princeton, NJ: Hosted by Robert Wood Johnson Foundation and the American Heart Association.

Reedy, J., & Krebs-Smith, S. M. (2010). Dietary sources of energy, solid fats, and added sugars among children and adolescents in the United States. *Journal of the American Dietetic Association, 110*, 1477–1484.

Rogers, R. (2012, July 15). Bitter fight over sugar: A councilman in Richmond leads an effort to tax sugary drinks. Rich foes line up against him. *Los Angeles Times.*

Roisman, H. (2013a, October 11). Deep in the heart of taxes, redux. *Telluride Daily Planet.*

Roisman, H. (2013b, November 1). Responding to the R-1 board. *Telluride Daily Planet.*

Ryan, C (1991). *Prime time activism: Media strategies for grassroots organizing.* Boston, MA: South End Press.

Samuels, B., & Glantz, S. A. (1991). The politics of local tobacco control. *JAMA: The Journal of the American Medical Association, 266*, 2110–2117.

Sasseen, J., Olmstead, K., & Mitchell, A. (2013). Digital: As mobile grows rapidly, the pressures on news intensify. In The Pew Center Project for Excellence in Journalism. *The state of the news media 2013: An annual report on American journalism.* Retrieved January 15, 2014, from http://stateofthemedia.org/2013/digital-as-mobile-grows-rapidly-the-pressures-on-news-intensify/

Scheufele, D., & Tewksbury, D. (2007). Framing, agenda setting, and priming: The evolution of three media effects models. *Journal of Communication, 57*, 9–20.

Smart Voter. (2012). *Measure O: Business license fee advisory measure – City of Richmond.* Retrieved March 18, 2014, from http://www.smartvoter.org/2012/11/06/ca/cc/meas/O/

Smith, C., & Ritterman, J. (2012, September 30). Point-counter point: Richmond measure N Soda Tax. *Halfway to Concord.*

Swisher, C. K., & Reese, S. D. (1992). The smoking and health issue in newspapers: Influence of regional economies, the tobacco institute and news objectivity. *Journalism & Mass Communication Quarterly, 69*, 987–1000. doi:10.1177/107769909206900417

Taddonio, B. (2013, November 1). The best offense is a good defense. *Telluride Daily Planet.*

US Census (2010). *American FactFinder – Community Facts.* Retrieved March 28, 2014, from http://factfinder2.census.gov/faces/nav/jsf/pages/community_facts.xhtml

Vartanian, L. R., Schwartz, M. B., & Brownell, K. D. (2007). Effects of soft drink consumption on nutrition and health: A systematic review and meta-analysis. *American Journal of Public Health, 97*, 667–675.

Velazquez, M. (2012a, July 23). El Monte Council to consider fiscal emergency, "sweet" tax for November ballot. *San Gabriel Valley Tribune.*

Velazquez, M. (2012b, October 8). El Monte to spend roughly $100,000 to place "soda tax" on special election ballot. *San Gabriel Valley Tribune.*

Velazquez, M. (2012c, September 6). Residents, business owners file arguments on El Monte ballot initiatives. *San Gabriel Valley Tribune.*

Wang, Y. C., Coxson, P., Shen, Y. M., Goldman, L., & Bibbins-Domingo, K. (2012). A penny-per-ounce tax on sugar-sweetened beverages would cut health and cost burdens of diabetes. *Health Affairs, 31*, 199–207. doi:10.1377/hlthaff.2011.0410

Welsh, J. A., Sharma, A. J., Grellinger, L., & Vos, M. B. (2011). Consumption of added sugars is decreasing in the United States. *American Journal of Clinical Nutrition, 94*, 726–734.

Whitney, S. (2012, May 16). Soda tax voted on to Richmond ballot. *Richmond Confidential.*

Wilkey, R. (2013, October 28). San Francisco soda tax proposed by city supervisor. *The Huffington Post.*

Woodward-Lopez, G., Kao, J., & Ritchie, L. (2010). To what extent have sweetened beverages contributed to the obesity epidemic? *Public Health Nutr, 14*, 499–509. doi: 10.1017/s1368980010002375

Yach, D., & Bialous, S. A. (2001). Junking science to promote tobacco. *American Journal of Public Health, 91*, 1745–1748. doi:10.2105/ajph.91.11.1745

Yanamadala, S., Bragg, M. A., Roberto, C. A., & Brownell, K. D. (2012). Food industry front groups and conflicts of interest: The case of Americans against food taxes. *Public Health Nutrition, 15*, 1331–1332.

Zingale, D. (2012, December 9). Gulp! The high cost of Big Soda's victory. *Los Angeles Times.*

'Big Food' and 'gamified' products: promotion, packaging, and the promise of fun

Charlene Elliott

Department of Communication and Culture, Faculty of Arts and Faculty of Kinesiology, University of Calgary, Calgary, Canada

The promise of 'fun' is an increasingly common strategy used by Big Food in the promotion of packaged products. *Gamification*, or 'making it fun', has been identified as a top consumer packaged goods trend for 2014, and is finding its way into the spectrum of packaged goods and target markets. Once solely the preserve of children's fare, fun is now applied to 'junk' food, 'healthy' food, snack food, 'adult' food, and 'kids' food. The rise and implications of such marketing has yet to be explored, and this article draws from the critical literature in food studies, current food marketing campaigns, and primary research from the trade press to map and critique 'fun' in association with food promotion. I argue that the promise of fun – while positioned as a playful, edible 'pause' in a hectic world – works to occlude some significant health, attitudinal and policy considerations related to the industrial diet. The seemingly lightweight focus on fun as a driver in food promotion promises a more embodied level of engagement than does a focus on nutritionism. However, 'fun' can simultaneously work to reconfigure relationships with food, increase consumption, and distance processed foodstuffs from issues of nutrients, as well as the non-communicable diseases associated with excessive consumption of highly processed fare.

In February 2014, the trade magazine *Food Navigator* reported on the growing success of Muller yogurt – a brand that is 'on pace' to achieve $100 million in annual retail sales in the United States (Watson, 2014). *Food Navigator's* interview with Chief Marketing Officer Barb Yehling was typical in the sense of her emphasis on the company's focus to provide 'irresistible products' that 'satisfy consumer desire'. Yet, Yehling's headline comment – 'Yogurt should be fun' (which was also the headline of the article) – is noteworthy. As Yehling explained, the fun imperative does not mean that Muller isn't healthy and delicious; it means that it is 'playful' and 'the focus is on fun' (Watson, 2014).

It might seem curious that 'fun' comprises the primary promotional message for a Greek yogurt aimed at adults. However, the promise of fun in food is an increasingly common strategy used by 'Big Food' in the promotion of packaged products. This article will suggest that the seemingly lightweight focus on 'fun' as a central driver in food promotion works to reconfigure relationships with food, increase consumption, and distance processed foodstuffs from issues of nutrients, as well as the non-communicable diseases associated with excessive consumption of highly processed fare.

Multinational giant PepsiCo, for example, has clustered the products comprising its $65 billion business into three Food Portfolios designed to satisfy the spectrum of consumer demands: the *Fun-for-You Portfolio* (comprised of Pepsi, Doritos, Cheetos, potato chips, and corn chips), a *Better-for-You Portfolio* (with baked potato chips, diet beverages, and granola bars), and a *Good-for-You Portfolio* (that includes instant oatmeal, orange juice, and cereal bars). Pearl Olives, launched in September 2013 as a healthy 'back-to-school snack' for children, has the tagline 'Fun at Your Fingertips' (www.pearlolives.com). (Advertisements encourage children to show off their 'olive fingers' by placing an olive on the tip of each finger.) General Mills' popular 'subscription snacking' service Nibblr (www.nibblrbox.com) delivers non-branded snack combinations (such as dried fruit, nuts and crackers) to offices and homes across the US. Subscription snacking is deemed to be the 'next generation business growth' by the company, and described by General Mills' marketing director Martin Abrams as delivering 'original and playful content' that gives subscribers 'a fun moment in their day' (Culliney, 2014b). Finally, market research company Datamonitor Consumer identifies the 'gamification' of products as a top consumer packaged goods trend for 2014. 'Gamification', otherwise known as 'making it fun', is touted as a key strategy for building engagement and loyalty in consumers, adults, and children alike (Hennessy, 2014).

The funning of food, I suggest, is a powerful, yet often overlooked, symbolic theme that characterizes contemporary food marketing. From PepsiCo's Fun-for-You product portfolio and subscription snacking to the trend of gamification, fun traverses the spectrum of packaged foods and target markets. Once solely the preserve of children's fare, fun is now applied to 'junk' food, 'healthy' food, snack food, 'adult' food, and children's food. The rise and unintended effects of such marketing has yet to be explored, and this article maps and critiques 'fun' in association with food promotion. Drawing from critical literature in food studies, policy papers/recommendations pertaining to food, and primary research from the trade press, I argue that the promise of fun – while positioned as a playful, edible 'pause' in a hectic world – works to occlude some significant health, attitudinal, and policy considerations related to the 'industrial diet' (Winson, 2013).

'Big Food' scholarship and typical packaged food marketing appeals

Impact of the multinational food industry on the diet

A growing body of scholarship critically examines the role of multinational food and beverage companies in relation to a host of socio-political and health problems. Nestle (2007, 2010), Simon (2006), Lang and Heasman (2004), Patel (2007), Winson (2013), Moss (2013), and Freudenberg (2014), among many others, have meticulously documented the different ways the food system (powerfully influenced by the food industry) has worked to promote corporate health over human health. It is no longer surprising to encounter arguments that describe how corporations contribute to the myriad health problems facing contemporary citizens. The food industry has indisputably transformed what we eat, how we eat it, and what we think of food (Patel, 2012). Awareness that the food industry's primary responsibility is to increase shareholder value means that consumers are constantly urged to buy more, not less food – often of dubious nutritional value (Nestle, 2007). Scholars have thus coined various terms to describe the resulting food environment as shaped by 'Big Food'. It has been labeled 'toxic'

(Brownell & Horgen, 2004), 'obesogenic' (Swinburn, Egger, & Raza, 1999) and an 'eat more' environment (Nestle & Nesheim, 2012) by public health advocates because of the ways that it promotes constant eating, typically of highly processed, junk food, and/or fast food. Some health researchers have suggested the need for an even more aggressive nomenclature that 'fits the risk' of the high-sugar, high-salt, and/or high-fat foods being sold to consumers: specifically, that such processed foods should be labeled 'pathogenic' foods, since they are 'likely to contribute to illness and premature death' (Campbell, Raine, & McLaren, 2012, p. 404). Other public health scholars have detailed how the 'corporate consumption complex', which promotes the 'hyperconsumption of products' and the selling of processed foods, is fundamentally in the business of 'manufacturing disease' (Freudenberg, 2014. Also see Kessler, 2009; Moss, 2013). Terms like 'industrial mass diet' further seek to draw attention to the political dimensions of diets, which reflect the material, political, and regulatory conditions of the industrial era, characterized by food commodity systems (Winson, 2013). Indeed, the somber tone of these terms describing the current food environment – toxic, obesogenic, pathogenic, industrial – communicate a type of caustic wasteland that is decidedly at odds with the fun eating promised by the food industry itself. Fun functions as a powerful diversion in the promotional messaging of processed foods. Unlike Type II diabetes, obesity, cardiovascular disease, and the range of non-communicable diseases associated with the processed food diet, fun is not a social or public health problem in need of solving.

The marketing of health

It is certainly not surprising that the food industry's promotional rhetoric is at odds with that of public health scholars. Popular food marketing claims like 'natural' and the increasing prominence of nutritionally enhanced and 'better-for-you' products in supermarkets (which foreground desirable components such as fiber, micronutrients, and probiotics) do little to communicate the negative impacts of consuming a highly processed food diet. Government-regulated nutrient content claims (such as 'excellent source of fibre') and diet-related health claims (such as 'a healthy diet low in saturated fat may reduce the risk of heart disease') popular with the food industry as marketing appeals remain quite distinct from the 'fun' applied to yogurt, olives, cheese, snack foods, junk foods, and many other adult foods and children's foods in the contemporary marketplace.

When it comes to the appeals typifying commercially packaged food products today 'nutri-speak' and 'nutritionism' dominate (Scrinis, 2013). Gyorgy Scrinis observes that 'nutri-speak' – the tendency to describe and evaluate the American diet using nutrient-level terms – has a long history, stretching back to the discovery of macronutrients in the mid-nineteenth century and vitamins in the early twentieth century (2013, pp. 36, 50–72). Scrinis traces how nutrition science and nutrition 'experts' have paved the way for the commodification of nutritionism, whereby corporations apply nutrient knowledge to sell food products. Nutritionism is often little more than 'nutritional façade', he argues (p. 8). This nutritional façade can be exemplified by Kellogg's Honey Smacks cereal, which prominently displays 'Good Source of Vitamin D' on the box, yet is 55.6% sugar by weight or Nature's Path Envirokidz Koala Crisp Cereal. Although 'organic', 'low sodium', and 'gluten free', EnviroKidz Koala Crisp cereal has the same percentage of sugar calories found in General Mills' marshmallow-filled Lucky Charms (both 40%) and a higher percentage of calories from sugar than

Kellogg's Pop Tarts (36%) (Elliott, 2012b, p. 271). In contrast to nutritionism, 'fun' is a relatively new – and profoundly significant – strategy used to market commercially packaged foods.

The point is that certain appeals have deep roots when it comes to promoting packaged foods. Such appeals include nutritionism, calories, fear, convenience, and pleasure – but fun (as will be argued) is a recent addition with cultural and health implications extending far beyond its playful trappings. While nutritionism has a long history (Scrinis, 2013), so, too, does the calorie. Many decades before the era of the 100-calorie snack pak (which transformed Nabisco Oreo 'Thin Crips' into a virtuous treat), Lulu Hunt Peters' 1918 diet book *Diet and Health, with Key to Calories* was a best seller in United States. Peters' book itemized foods in 100-calorie servings in order to help image-conscious consumers manage their weight (Scrinis, 2013, pp. 50–51). Levenstein's (2012) history of American food fears draws attention to a different, equally prominent concern picked up by food manufacturers in the aid of selling products: germs. In particular, Levenstein traces how industrialization of the food supply created consumer preoccupation with the dangers lurking in food (via germs, contaminants) that food processors could capitalize on in promoting packaged goods. Packaging, such as Kellogg's 1914 advertisement for its 'waxtite package', was advertised as protection against 'contamination by germs' (2012, p. 12). The H.J. Heinz Company similarly labeled its jarred pickles as products offering 'the exemplification of quality' (with the 'quality' referring to sanitization) to set it apart from the competition (p. 12). Beyond this, the promotion of packaged foods for its convenience – as a type of 'liberation' from the burden and drudgery of cooking – became a relentless advertising message to American women in the 1950s, which aimed to normalize the purchase of packaged products (Levenstein, 1993; Shapiro, 2004). Even a focus on the pleasure of food, often marketed with indulgence products (e.g. artisanal cheese, premium ice cream, premium chocolate) is categorically different from the 'funning' of food, of the framing of food as a vehicle of entertainment.

Food marketing and the rise of fun

Fun and children's food

In his analysis of contemporary child-oriented food marketing, Daniel Cook observes that fun food 'succinctly denotes a food item or category as belonging foremost to children and to a children's world' (Cook, 2005, p. 20). However, this has not always been the case. Historically, the dominant cultural attitude (in the United States and Canada, at least) was antithetical to fun in connection with food. At the turn of the nineteenth century, the notion of 'food fun' was verboten. As American pediatrician Luther Emmett Holt dictated to mothers in his manual *The Proper Care and Feeding of Children,* 'young children [age 4–10] should not be allowed to play with their food, nor should the habit be formed of amusing or diverting them while eating' (1894/1916, p. 147). This message received wide audience in light of the book's 78 print runs, 28 editions, and numerous translations in the decades that followed. Holt was America's most prominent child-rearing expert for nearly half a century, until the emergence of the highly popular Dr. Spock whose best-selling book (subsequently translated into 39 languages with more than 50 million copies sold) (Sealander, 2005, p. 172) similarly suggested that child feeding was not to be an extension of the playroom. While Spock does not directly engage with food play, he is emphatic that children should not be persuaded to eat via acts or bribes by parents, which transform mealtime and the singular act of eating into 'an hour's exhausting vaudeville' (Spock, 1946, p. 356). Games are to occur beyond, not within, the confines of eating, he affirms (pp. 358–360).

It was the recognition of the child as a valuable market in the 1930s – what Cook deems a turning point in the 'institutional adjudication of the child consumer' (2004, p. 2) – that first opened the doors for connecting play with food. Not only was this the decade that department and dry goods stores started to physically segregate children's merchandise in their retail spaces (i.e. to create separate departments for children) in order to sell to 'the mother through the child' (Cook, 2004, p. 50); equally important was seizing the child's attention and recognizing his or her viewpoint. *Pediocularity,* seeing with children's eyes or with their perspective in mind, became increasingly relevant to merchants and marketers seeking to move products (2004, p. 67). As the trade magazine *Printer's Ink Monthly* advised its readership in 1932, children should have specially designed packages, since what appeals to adults does not necessarily appeal to children (2004, p. 74). *Printer's Ink Monthly* also suggested 'story book food' as a way to target both the parent and the child. The magazine acknowledged that products like Animal Crackers 'are really only cookies made in the shape of animals' but that such story book foods work to increase sales by targeting both the parent and the child (quoted in Cook, 2004, p. 73).

Story book food stood as implicit acknowledgment that children's food needs could be different from those of adults for commercial purposes. Extending the 'story book' theme to food suggested a different type of need (distinct from calories or nutrition) and a different type of pleasure, distinct from taste or the more sophisticated, adult-oriented concerns pertaining to aesthetics. It was this recognition of the child as a choosing subject/consumer that first prompted food manufacturers to target them directly. Cream of Wheat, for instance, was one of the first advertisers to sponsor a children's radio program, a 15-minute musical entertainment show titled the *Cream of Wheat Menagerie,* which first aired in December 1928 (Asquith, 2011, pp. 104–110). *Cream of Wheat Menagerie* engaged the child listener with stories, fairy tales and the 'Musical Menagerie' (animals who played musical instruments), while reminding children to consume the cereal. Rapid growth in children's radio programming ensued: between 1928 and 1934, New York City radio stations launched over 75 children's commercial programs. Food advertisers sponsored more than half of these shows (2011, p. 107). In 1945, cereal maker Kellogg distinguished itself from its competition by being the first manufacturer to place a prize right into the box. Kellogg's offered children the 'exciting prize' of a tin pin-back button in PEP cereal. The buttons came in series (including five series of comic characters with 18 different buttons in each set), and early radio advertisements urged children to 'eat more of that super delicious whole wheat flake cereal so you get more prizes' (PEP Vintage, 1945). However, even though these food manufacturers were targeting children, there was nothing particularly 'fun' about the actual products. Cream of Wheat and PEP whole-wheat flake cereal were far removed from the cartoon characters, 'fun' shapes and colorful marshmallows often associated with the child-targeted cereals of today.

In the popular Canadian women's magazine *Chatelaine,* the first advertisement that literally linked packaged food with fun appeared in February 1939. It was for Kellogg, which presented packaged cereal as the solution to the troubles encountered by the modern housewife. Along with the claim that 'modern days demands modern breakfasts' (represented by Kellogg boxed cereals), the advertisement showed the image of a girl sitting at the kitchen table, delighted because her mother 'chose for her the cereal [that's] FUN to eat'. 'Little Anne' reinforces fun food's significance by calling out

'Mommy, these Krispies are <u>Fun!</u>' (Chatelaine, 'Rice Krispies' 1939, p. 53). Fun is not a dominant trope at this time, however. Advertisements related to children's eating are, instead, primarily focused on their energy needs (e.g. Crown Corn Syrup advertised as providing 'quick, needed energy' for children, *Chatelaine,* 1940). In July 1954, Kellogg re-emphasized the 'real fun' children can have choosing from Kellogg's variety package of single-serving cereals (Chatelaine, 1954, p. 45). This fun theme resurfaced several months later in an advertisement for Kellogg's Rice Krispies, which affirms that the cereal's 'Snap! Crackle! Pop' sounds 'tell you how crisp they are and how much fun they are for breakfast' (Chatelaine, 1954). By 1967, 'fun' became the headline appeal in an advertisement for Lipton Cowboy Beef Soup Mix, which embraced the story book food recommendation *Printer's Ink* magazine made roughly three decades earlier. 'Fun's on' announced the advertisement, which explained that the noodles were shaped like 'horses, stars, six guns and boots' (Chatelaine, 1967).

Although the concept developed slowly, 'fun' in association with children's food became increasingly prevalent. McDonald's applied the idea to fast food by introducing the Happy Meal into its US national menu in 1979. This well-known children's meal came in colorful box adorned with games, jokes and puzzles, and with a toy. It was explicitly advertised on television as 'food and fun in a box' (McDonalds, 1979). Indeed, it is worth noting that the ongoing popularity of this children's meal has allowed McDonald's to lay claim to being the largest toy distributor in the world ('Industry News,' 2011, p. 9). Moreover, despite the ongoing debate over the ethics of manipulating children to request fast food in order to get a toy, McDonald's has defended its 'fun food' approach. When McDonald's launched its Ice Age Happy Meal 'event' in the US market in 2009 with a collection of eight toys from the popular children's movie, McDonald's global chief marketing officer pointed to the Ice Age-themed wrapping found on packaged McDonald's Apple Dippers and its low fat white and chocolate milk. He affirmed that the Happy Meal event 'reach[ed] kids in a fun and responsible way' ('Fun Heats Up,' 2009).

By the late 1990s and early 2000s, the concept of fun in association with children's food was being explicitly promoted by the trade press and wholly embraced food manufacturers. '*The fun starts here*' became the umbrella theme of Kraft Foods' 1999 campaign to promote its Post cereals to children. It formed a core part of the company's plan to 'leverage its presweetened cereals under the Post kids banner' and to demonstrate its 'commitment to innovation with its kid-targeted cereal brands' (Thompson, 1999, p. 19). Kellogg similarly announced it was 'bringing fun into the cereal aisle' (Kellogg Company, 1999), and Kraft Foods launched Lunchables Fun Snacks with a US $25 million campaign and the slogan 'some snacks have all the fun' (Thompson, 2001, p. 45). 'Fun food' proliferated throughout the supermarket, with hundreds of products spanning every product category (Elliott, 2008). Notable about these supermarket foods is that they are 'regular' foods (such as cheese, crackers, cereals, yogurts, frozen meats, etc.) that have been redesigned to appeal to children. Such appeals often include direct claims or allusions to 'fun' on the package, cartoon iconography pointedly targeted to children, tie-ins with children's television programs, merchandise or films, the foregrounding of unusual shapes, colors or flavors, and/or puzzles or games targeted at children (Elliott, 2008, 2012a).

'Fun' in these packaged foods is not merely communicated by cartoon characters on the container and unique shapes. Fun is literally built into the product names and stated on the packages themselves. Since the late 1990s, 'fun' supermarket foods have included Parkay's Fun Squeeze margarine, Black Diamond Funcheez processed cheese,

Eggo Fun Pix waffles, Nabisco's Oreo Fun Stix (promoted as a 'fun alternative to breakfast cereal'), SunRype's FunBites fruit snacks, and Schneider's Lunch Mate Fun Kits that invited children to build their own lunchtime treats out of cookies, icing, and sprinkles. In the marketplace of children's foods, packages affirm the food's 'assorted fun colours', and 'fun flavours' or its 'fun shapes'. Edibles are also framed as a *gateway* to fun with packages underscoring the fun experience of consuming the product. Fruit snacks and cookie packages claim that they're 'fun to eat!' Kool-Aid drink crystals instruct consumers to 'mix up some fun!' and squeezable yogurt tubes claim to be 'a lot of fun' (Elliott, 2012a). Even products designed to leverage consumer interest in health embrace the concept of fun. In fact, a content analysis of 354 foods targeted at children in the Canadian supermarket revealed that the products promoted as 'better-for-you' were more likely to reference 'fun' on the package than 'regular' child targeted foods (Elliott, 2012b, p. 275). This study found that 29% of 'better-for-you' products made a direct statement about 'fun' somewhere on the package, compared to 23% of 'regular' products. When over one in every five packaged food products analyzed literally references 'fun', it seems reasonable to suggest that 'fun' has been embraced as a desirable marketing strategy.

Recent examples of this include Pearl Olives, marketed to children with the 'Fun at Your Fingertips' tag line and Disney Corporation's Disney Foodles and Disney Flavorz. Disney Foodles are advertised as 'combo packs' of fruits, vegetables, dips, and cheese in 'fun' shaped trays. Disney Flavorz are branded sliced apples infused with different flavors, such as the Princess pack, where the apples are the 'flavor' of Strawberry with Vanilla Cream. Its advertising copy claims that 'Flavorz Makes Apple Eating Fun' (Disney Flavorz, 2013). Disney Foodles and Flavorz extends the company's health-food promotions, which started with its 2006 launch of the Disney Garden line in which Disney-themed stickers appeared on produce ranging from apples to avocadoes (McDevitt, 2009). By 2009, Disney offered over 250 products in its lineup and also introduced Disney-branded eggs in two US states (Disney taking bite, 2009). Each eggshell came stamped with a Disney character (e.g. Mickey Mouse, Donald Duck, Tigger, Buzz Lightyear), and the eggs were advertised on American television as 'Great tasting, nutritious, and fun, too!'

Beyond children's food: Adults as the new audience for fun

'Fun' is linked to children's commercially produced food. However, the food industry's mandate to increase shareholder value leads to an ongoing push for new growth opportunities and marketing innovations. Part of this innovation can currently be seen in the creeping application of 'fun' to food outside of the (industry-created) category of 'kids' food'. Alongside the 'yogurt should be fun' claim of Muller yogurt and PepsiCo's 'Fun-for-You' product portfolio (which does not primarily target children), are also chocolate bars marketed in 'fun' sizes, packaged cupcake mixes called *Fun-da-Middles* advertised as 'a fun introduction to baking for millennial generation moms' and a series of marketing campaigns for 'fun' cereals aimed at adults. Nestle's new Toffee Crisp cereal, introduced to the UK market in February 2014, targets adults over age 35. It is discussed in the trade magazine *Food Navigator* as an 'exciting opportunity' that equally gives adults the chance to 'eat something that is still a bit of fun' (Culliney, 2014a). General Mills initiated a national cereal lovers campaign across the US in October 2013 to 'raise enthusiasm for the cereal category' and to remind Americans that, 'At the heart of it, cereal is all about fun' (Culliney, 2013b). Finally, market research studies on consumer trends indicate that 'fun' is a growth opportunity for snack makers targeting women. Reported in *Food Nagivator's* 'Breaking News on Food & Beverage Development' section is the finding that, in the US and Europe, 'fun' (not health) is the number three motivator for women snackers – ranked after indulgence and personal space (Culliney, 2013a). Consumer market research firm Mintel supports this trend toward snacking fun with its 2012 report on the US $13.6 billion 'Chips, Pretzels and Corn Snacks' market, which Mintel frames as a popular category and a 'fairly reliable revenue stream'. Its report provides insight to how the snacking industry develops and markets products that meet 'consumers' desire for fun and taste' while 'balancing this against a growing interest in eating better' (Mintel, 2012). Mintel also highlights Wonderful Pistachios as exemplar of the marketing strategy promoting the 'theme of fun' in its January 2014 report on the US market for *Chips, Popcorn, Nuts, and Dips*. This is currently a US $21.8 billion market (Mintel, 2014).

'Big Food', health, and the significance of fun

With this 'new' audience for fun, it is the concept of gamification that is worth considering, the marketing strategy of 'making it fun' (Hennessy, 2014). Many categories of processed foods do not fall under the fun theme. However, its presence in snack foods, ready-to-eat cereals, yogurts, olives, nuts, packaged cupcake mixes, and confectionary suggest that 'fun' is of increasing value. Fun is a significant strategy Big Food uses to increase consumption of its products for several reasons. First, PepsiCo's 'Fun-for-You' portfolio comprised of regular Pepsi, Mountain Dew, Doritos, Cheetos, Lay's, Tostitos (and other brands) is described on PepsiCo's website as 'food and beverages making life more fun for people' (http://www.pepsico.com/Brands/BrandExplorer#fun-for-you). Identifying such brands as 'Fun-for-You' allows PespiCo to sidestep a more obvious critique, namely that they are 'Bad-for-You' or 'junk' foods. Fun has positive connotations: attempts to deny an individual's right to 'fun' often comes with resistance (e.g. consider the 'nanny state' criticisms that frequently arise when public health advocates seek to influence consumer food choices). Fun also redirects attention away from the nutritional qualities of food: fun and nutrition are completely separate categories. This said, the increasing prevalence of 'healthier' foods promoting the 'fun' theme reveals its desirability – and its normalization – as an attribute of food. Finally, 'fun' is used to propel product growth and sales. For instance, 'fun' sized chocolate bars provide a new angle on a commonplace product.

The reclassification of packaged/processed fare as 'fun' requires some consideration. As a classificatory schemata, fun adds another dimension to the evaluation of food. To the questions of 'is it healthy?', 'is it tasty?', 'is it organic/free range/GMO free?' (etc.) that consumers might ask of their food, this promotional strategy suggests that people should also be asking: 'is it fun?'. Fun has become an additional layer to food – and the *funning* of food (which is about entertainment) is quite different from appreciating its aesthetic qualities, taste, or origins. Scholarly research on food classification has suggested that individuals attribute three core dimensions to food: functional, concrete-descriptive, and affective (Young, 2000). *Functional* refers to a culturally recognized 'function' that distinguishes foods from each other (such as 'healthy'/'good for you' – 'unhealthy'/'bad for you'; snack/meal; breakfast/lunch/dinner). *Concrete/descriptive* refers to perceptual distinctions (such as shape or size, or crunchiness, sweetness, etc.). *Affective* dimensions pertain to the emotional quality experienced by individuals themselves (such as like/dislike) (Young, 2000). What is noteworthy about the 'fun' appeal promoted by Big Food is that it covers two of these three classificatory schemes: the functional (i.e. 'fun for you') as well as the affective. Fun is an experiential state, defined as something intended purely for amusement. To suggest that fun is the primary motivator for eating pistachios reconfigures relationships with food. Framing sugary soda, potato chips and cheezies as 'Fun-for-You' distances low-nutrient, highly processed foods from the negative health consequences of their consumption. Indeed, some trade magazines have so fully embraced these functional and affective dimensions that they suggest that fun is fundamental to food. A recent *Food Navigator* article on dairy trends observes the steady decline in milk consumption by children over the past three decades and queries: "So how can food marketers make milk fun again?" (Watson, 2013). Implicit, here, is the assumption that milk was fun in the first place, and that its muting has resulted in declining consumption. The proposed solution is to 'fun-it-up' by adding 'healthy' Moo Mixer syrups (which contain stevia extract, sugar, and cultured dextrose) to transform milk into Twerple Purple, Moolectric Blue, Inky Pinky, and other colorful 'flavors' (Watson, 2013). Moo Mixers Syrups' CEO affirms that funning is framed as a 'great way to get kids to drink more milk'. More important to this framework is the way that the absence of fun becomes the justification for food manipulation.

Repositioning fun as an affective dimension of food raises some interesting implications for our long-held and reductive mode of evaluating food: nutritionism. Scrinis explains that engaging with food at the nutrient level is 'a more abstract way of encountering food since it involves a less embodied level of engagement' (2013, p. 27). I suggest that the food industry has subtly introduced a strategy that fundamentally counters the 'less embodied level of engagement' found in nutritionism. Fun, premised on the experience of consumption, brings the concrete 'experience' of food to the foreground.

The positive association of fun, coupled with its innocuous nature, means that some possible unintended consequences get overlooked with regards to the food-as-fun theme. Research with preschoolers suggests that very young children will consume 50% more vegetables when they are given 'catchy' names like X-ray-Vision carrots because they think they will be more fun to eat (Wansink, Just, & Smith, 2011). Increasing consumption through the promise of fun might be a positive outcome for young children who dislike vegetables. However, if fun actually prompts individuals to eat more – which certainly seems to be the premise found in the trade magazines – it is problematic for public health. Public health scholars already lament that we reside in an 'Eat More' environment (Nestle & Nesheim, 2012). Adding extra encouragement to eat more through the appeal to fun in an already 'Eat More' environment may prove excessive (particularly in light of the obesity epidemic).

Fun is strategic marketing for Big Food because the very sentiment of fun distracts from questions of calories, nutrients, and origin while promoting consumption. Arguably, fun is a powerful promotional strategy in what Winson (2013) deems the 'industrial diet' – a diet characterized predominantly by nutrient-poor 'pseudo foods' that (historically) became acceptable due to successful mass communication/mass advertising campaigns that foregrounded the desirable aspects of processed foodstuffs. The upside of fun is that, while it might comprise part of the 'pseudo-foods' in the industrial diet, 'fun' does not sound industrial in the least. The remarkable part about the fun theme is its emergence, not only in 'adult' foods, but also in less-processed fare – which suggests that producers of actual 'good for you' edibles (olives, pistachios) feel compelled to echo the marketing strategies of purveyors of 'pseudo food'. This is particularly striking in light of heightened consumer interest in health, minimally processed foods and/or 'better-for-you' products.

Considerations on the trend towards fun and on policy

Fun, I have suggested, is an increasingly prominent strategy used by the food industry in the promotion of packaged products. Applying this unusual attribute to food is rather new, starting with children's fare and only very recently fanning outward to target older age groups. Despite its lightweight connotations, fun as a food marketing strategy is also remarkably complex. Gamification in children's food has, to date, pertained to shapes, fun names, or unusual tastes, and the ways that processed foods might act as a gateway to fun through associations with cartoons, interactivity, or even transgressiveness. From its origins as story book food (cookies shaped into animals) and Rice Krispies (that make sounds, which cereal does not typically do), to yogurt tubes designed to be squirted directly in the mouth (negating the need for a spoon) or Disney Princess Apples that taste like strawberries and vanilla cream, the 'fun' in children's food is often about foregrounding its entertaining or interactive properties. Products that are *not* altered (in taste, or shape, or color) may emphasize transgressiveness as a pathway to food fun: putting an olive on each fingertip is 'fun' because it transgresses cultural protocols and adult manners (i.e. that is not the way that olives should be eaten). Overall, gamification in children's food is generally about reconfiguring the food itself or how it is eaten in order to emphasize fun. It asks children to approach or treat food as entertainment or as a game, and not as food. The extension of 'fun' into adult food promotion, however, is less clearly demarcated. Subscription snacking emphasizes variety and a pause in a workday, the notion of 'fun sized' chocolate bars are often advertised as items that can be consumed without guilt or fear of gaining weight,[1] and campaigns to encourage adults to view yogurt or cereals or 'junk' food as 'fun' suggests a different kind of attitude toward food compared to child-targeted fare. Nothing in particular about Muller yogurt (targeted at adults) makes it 'fun' beyond the claim by the CMO that its yogurt is playful and primarily about fun. PepsiCo's Fun-for-You portfolio and 'fun sized' chocolate bars similarly encourage an *attitude* about food – an attitude that encourages adults to eat without worrying about calories, nutritional profile, origins, etc. While child-oriented food is more about entertainment through food and adult-oriented 'fun' is more about an attitude toward eating, both sidestep issues of nutrition, calories, politics, and health. The result is a significant gap between what public health experts ask consumers to consider about food and what marketers advertise as important. Fun poses a challenge to public health because it falls outside the purview of policy, yet powerfully reconfigures ideas of what consumers should consider when they approach food. Policy focuses on nutritionism. Gamification focuses on the experiential dimensions of food (and often experiential dimensions that are external to the food itself). While nutritionism and gamification are mutually exclusive, both are tremendously important when it comes to consumer attitudes and considerations around eating. Combatting an 'eat more' environment strictly at the level of nutrition is a losing proposition, and future research should remain attentive to how 'Big Food' marketing strategies introduce new issues into the field of public health.

Disclosure statement

The author has no conflicts of interest to disclose. The author has no financial interest or benefit arising from the direct applications of their research.

Acknowledgements

This study was supported by the Canada Research Chairs program, and the BMO Research Prize on Healthy Living. The author would also like to acknowledge the Calgary Institute for the Humanities (CIH), where she is currently Scholar in Residence.

Note

1. Thank you to an anonymous reviewer for this point, and also the interesting observation that in public health terms, 'fun sized' chocolate bars could be understood as 'harm minimization' (i.e. eat a 'fun' sized chocolate bar rather than a whole bar).

References

Asquith, K. (2011). *Aren't they keen? Early children's food advertising and the emergence of the brand-loyal child consumer* (Unpublished Dissertation). University of Western Ontario, London, Ontario.

Brownell, K., & Horgen, K. B. (2004). *Food fight: The inside story of the food industry, America's obesity crisis and what we can do about it*. New York, NY: Contemporary Books.

Campbell, N., Raine, K., & McLaren, L. (2012). "Junk Foods," "Treats," or "Pathogenic Foods"? A call for changing nomenclature to fit the risk of today's diets. *Canadian Journal of Cardiology, 28*, 403–404.

Cook, D. (2004). *The commodification of childhood*. Durham: Duke University Press.

Cook, D. (2005, August 12). *How food consumer 'the child' in the corporate landscape of fun: Commerce, agency, and culture*. Paper presented at the annual meeting of the American Sociological Association, Marriott Hotel, Loews Philadelphia Hotel, Philadelphia, PA. Retrieved from http://www.allacademic.com/meta/p19102_index.html

Culliney, K. (2013a, June 19). Women want indulgence and health in snacks ... scrap that stereotype, says Canadean. *Food Navigator – USA*.

Culliney, K. (2013b, October 16). General Mills wants to liven up cereal: 'It's part of the American pop culture'. *Food Navigator – USA*. Retrieved from http://www.foodnavigator-usa.com/Manufacturers/General-Mills-wants-to-liven-up-cereal-It-s-part-of-the-American-pop-culture

Culliney, K. (2014a, January 21). Adult fun: Nestle extends toffee crisp chocolate bar into cereal. *Food Navigator – USA*. Retrieved from http://www.bakeryandsnacks.com/Manufacturers/Adult-fun-Nestle-extends-Toffee-Crisp-chocolate-bar-into-cereal

Culliney, K. (2014b, January 7). General mills: Next generation growth is in subscription snacking. *Food Navigator – USA*. Retrieved from http://www.foodnavigator-usa.com/Manufacturers/General-Mills-Next-generation-growth-is-in-subscription-snacking

Disney Flavorz. (2013). *Crunch pak makes apple eating fun with flavorz*. Retrieved from http://www.crunchpak.com/products/flavorz/

Disney taking bite out of new foods. (2009). *Licensing Letter, 33*, 2.

Elliott, C. (2008). Marketing fun foods: A profile and analysis of supermarket food messages targeted at children. *Canadian Public Policy, 34*, 259–273.

Elliott, C. (2012a). Packaging fun: Analysing supermarket food messages targeted at children. *Canadian Journal of Communication, 37*, 303–318.

Elliott, C. (2012b). Packaging Health: Examining "better-for-you" foods targeted at children. *Canadian Public Policy, 38*, 265–281.

Freudenberg, N. (2014). *Lethal but legal. Corporations, consumption and protecting public health*. New York, NY: Oxford University Press.

Fun heats up at McDonald's(R) with launch of the coolest global happy meal event in ages – twentieth century fox's 'ice age: Dawn of the dinosaurs'. (2009, June 18). *Canada NewsWire*. [Ottawa].

Hennessy, M. (2014, February 5). Drinkable veggies, smart packaging, 'gamified products': Datamonitor's 10 CPG trends. *Food Navigator – USA*. Retrieved from http://www.foodnavigator-usa.com/Markets/Drinkable-veggies-smart-packaging-gamified-products-Datamonitor-s-10-CPG-trends

Holt, L. E. (1894/1916). *The care and feeding of children: A catechism for the use of mothers and children's nurses*. New York, NY: D. Appleton.

Industry news & notes. (2011). *Journal of Property Management, 76*, 9.

Kellogg Company brings fun back into the cereal aisle with Sesame Street Mini-Beans inpack premium offer. (1999, December 8). *Business Wire*. Retrieved August 2009, from http://findarticles.com/p/articles/mi_m0EIN/is_1999_Dec_8/ai_58079654

Kessler, D. (2009). *The end of overeating: Taking control of the insatiable American appetite*. Emmaus: Rodale.

Lang, T., & Heasman, M. (2004). *Food wars the global battle for mouths, minds and market*. New York, NY: Routledge.

Levenstein, H. (1993). *Paradox of plenty: A social history of eating in modern America*. Oxford: Oxford University Press.

Levenstein, H. (2012). *Fear of food*. Chicago, IL: University of Chicago Press.

McDevitt, C. (2009, May 3). A Hannah Montana banana? Disney's brand goes healthy. *The Washington Post*. G02.

McDonalds. (1979). "Introducing the happy meal" (television commercial). *The Museum of Classic Chicago Television*. Retrieved from http://www.youtube.com/watch?v=9qAfN_5ZIbM

Mintel. (2012, January). *Chips, pretzels and corn snacks – US*. London: Author. Retrieved from http://store.mintel.com/chips-pretzels-and-corn-snacks-us-january-2012?cookie_test=true

Mintel. (2014, January). *Chips, popcorn, nuts, and dips – US*. London: Author.

Moss, M. (2013). *Salt, sugar, fat: How the food giants hooked us*. Toronto: Random House.

Nestle, M. (2007). *Food politics: How the food industry influences nutrition and health*. Berkeley: University of California Press.

Nestle, M. (2010). *Safe food: The politics of food safety*. Berkeley: University of California Press.

Nestle, M., & Nesheim, M. (2012). *Why calories count: From science to politics*. Berkeley: University of California Press.

Patel, R. (2007). *Stuffed and starved: The hidden battle for the world's food system*. Toronto: Harper Perennial.

Patel, R. (2012, February 6). Abolish the food industry. *The Atlantic*. Retrieved from http://www.theatlantic.com/health/archive/2012/02/abolish-the-food-industry/252502

PEP Vintage. (1945). Retrieved from http://www.oldtimeradiodownloads.com/mp3/commercials/Vintage%20Radio%20Commercials/Vintage%20Commercials%20Kellogs%20Pep.mp3

Scrinis, G. (2013). *Nutritionism: The science and politics of dietary advice*. New York, NY: Columbia University Press.

Sealander, J. (2005). Perpetually malnourished? Diet, health, and America's young in the twentieth century In C.K. Warsh & V. Strong-Boag (Eds.), *Children's health in historical perspective* (pp. 161–189). Ontario, Canada: Wilfred Laurier University Press.

Shapiro, L. (2004). *Something from the oven: Reinventing dinner in 1950s America*. New York, NY: Penguin.

Simon, M. (2006). *Appetite for profit: How the food industry undermines our health and how to fight back*. New York, NY: Nation Books.

Spock, B. (1946). *The common sense book of baby and child care*. New York, NY: Duell, Sloan and Pearce.

Swinburn, B., Egger, G., & Raza, F. (1999). Dissecting obesogenic environments: The development and application of a framework for identifying and prioritizing environmental interventions for obesity. *Preventive Medicine, 29*, 563–570.

Thompson, S. (1999). Kraft-y promo: Post gives coins for 'comb'. *Advertising Age, 70*, 19.

Thompson, S. (2001). Kraft launches Lunchables for *snack* attacks. *Advertising Age, 72*, 45.

Wansink, B., Just, D., & Smith, L. (2011). What is in a name? Giving descriptive names to vegetables increases lunchroom sales. *JNEB, 43*(S1).

Watson, E. (2013, November 11). Moo mixer syrups CEO: Want your kids to drink milk instead of juice and soda? Try this .... *Food Navigator – USA*. Retrieved from http://www.foodnavigator-usa.com/People/Moo-Mixers-Syrups-CEO-Want-your-kids-to-drink-milk-instead-of-juice-and-soda-Try-this

Watson, E. (2014, February 10). In conversation with Muller Quaker Dairy as Muller brand approaches $100m in US: 'Yogurt should be fun'. *Food Navigator – USA*. Retrieved from http://www.foodnavigator-usa.com/Manufacturers/In-conversation-with-Muller-Quaker-Dairy-as-Mueller-brand-approaches-100 m-in-US-Yogurt-should-be-fun

Winson, A. (2013). *The industrial diet: The degradation of food and the struggle for healthy eating*. Toronto: UBC Press.

Young, B. M. (2000). Children's categorization of foods. *International Journal of Advertising, 19*, 495–508.

Magazine advertisements

Chatelaine – February 1939, July 1954, November 1954, February 1967.

Food as pharma: marketing nutraceuticals to India's rural poor

Alice Street

Social Anthropology, University of Edinburgh, Edinburgh, UK

This commentary sketches out the politics of the expansion of affordable, fast-moving nutraceutical products into rural India, with a focus on fortified foods and beverages. It examines the relationships between industry, government and humanitarian organisations that are being forged alongside the development of markets for nutraceuticals; the production of evidence and the harnessing of science to support nutraceutical companies' claims; the ways in which nutraceuticals are being marketed and distributed in rural areas; and the concepts of health and well-being that are being promulgated through those marketing campaigns. Lastly, it asks what kinds of impact fast-moving nutraceuticals are likely to have on the lives of India's rural poor. It concludes by questioning how smooth a transition to nutraceutical consumption Big Food marketing strategies can really facilitate and how readily low-income families seeking to feed their families and safeguard health will actually adopt concepts of wellness and internalise micro-nutrient associated risks.

Introduction

In 2009, GlaxoSmithKline began test marketing an affordable brand of Horlicks™, its ubiquitous malt-based drink, to be sold in 2.5 rupee sachets in villages across Andhra Pradesh in South India. In marketing the product, which it called Asha™ (hope, in Hindi), GlaxoSmithKline claimed it would provide poor rural consumers with an alternative to local cereal mixes of what they call 'uncertain quality', such as finger millet malt. In 2011, PepsiCo India launched a new salty biscuit product called Lehar Iron Chusti™, which it rolled out across Andhra Pradesh in 2 rupee packets, alongside a major education campaign on iron deficiency for women and teenagers. At the same time, in neighbouring Orissa, Coca-Cola was launching Vitingo™, a new sachet-based orange-flavoured drink fortified with 12 vitamins and minerals that it promoted as helping to combat blindness, anemia and other common diseases, in collaboration with a local NGO and self-help group.

These are all examples of what industry and marketing groups refer to as nutraceuticals: nutritionally fortified or engineered foods, beverages or supplements that are marketed for their health-giving properties. In recent years, Indian economists and market research agencies have championed the Indian nutraceuticals market as a potential engine of growth. With current growth rates exceeding 18% and market forecasts of a fivefold increase by 2020, nutraceuticals are celebrated as the most successful sector of the food and pharmaceuticals market (IKON Marketing Consultants, 2013; Indian Business News Agency, 2012). In 2010, revenues from the Indian nutraceutical industry were estimated at US $ 2 Billion (Frost & Sullivan, 2011, p. 5). By 2017, they are expected to reach US $ 4.2 billion (Techsi Research, 2013). The potential for expansion is deemed to be vast, with 'an envisaged latent market of 148 million customers' (Ernst & Young, 2012, p. 25).

Until recently, the nutraceutical industry had concentrated on responding to the rise in obesity and lifestyle diseases in India by marketing more expensive, higher margin products to India's aspirant middle class. Marketing consultants celebrate this population as having a growing awareness of health and lifestyle diseases, rising disposable incomes and, increasingly, a 'self-care ethos' that is associated with a demand for preventative healthcare products. To market analysts, food and beverage companies appear to be dividing their urban portfolio into complementary segments of health and wellness on the one hand and indulgence on the other (Gupta, 2009). Health and wellness products include sports beverages, diabetic foods and child health products. GlaxoSmithKline's Horlicks™ is seen as the market leader in this area, with diversification into 'Standard', 'Women's' and 'Children's' ranges, and securing 50% of the fortified beverage market in 2012. Horlicks™ is now the second-biggest selling beverage in India after bottled water and has double the sales figures of Coca-Cola and Pepsi combined.

But with intense competition in the urban sector, the focus of both domestic and multinational companies is now moving to the design of affordable nutraceutical goods for consumers at the 'bottom of the pyramid'; Indians who live on less than $2 a day (Prahalad, 2009). This is a largely rural population whose anticipated purchasing power is based on an economy of speed and scale rather than the size of individual incomes. Where the penetration rate of nutraceuticals in urban areas is 22.51%, in rural areas it is currently only 6.32%. For the growing nutraceutical industry and those seeking to make new acquisitions in this area, this presents a huge 'latent market' that could ultimately account for a third of the market scope (IKON Marketing Consultants, 2013).

The migration of the nutraceuticals industry into rural markets has seen the industry shift away from the claim that their products can prevent non-communicable diseases associated with urban working lifestyles, such as diabetes, cardiovascular disorders and cancers, and towards the claim that products specifically designed for the rural poor can tackle child malnutrition and save vulnerable lives. Such claims are couched in a language of humanitarianism and focused on a target that the food industry increasingly shares with the international development sector: micronutrient deficiency, its long-term health implications and its national and global economic cost.

Today, India's 'double burden' of obesity and malnutrition is a double opportunity. With the rise of micronutrient deficiency as a development problem, an international consensus has emerged around the corporate laboratory and marketing agency as the solution (Kimura, 2013). Where government food programs in India have failed to address rural malnutrition, it is anticipated that Big Food, with its scientific, marketing and distribution capacities can succeed. Selling nutraceuticals to the rural poor, according to governments; the food industry, a global community of market consultancy agencies and accountancy firms; and the global development community, is a clear case of 'doing well by doing good'.

This commentary sketches out the politics of the expansion of affordable, fast-moving[1] nutraceutical products into rural India, with a focus on fortified foods and beverages. It examines the relationships between industry, government and humanitarian organisations that are being forged alongside the development of markets for nutraceuticals; the production of evidence and the harnessing of science to support nutraceutical companies' claims; the ways in which nutraceuticals are being marketed and distributed in rural areas; and the concepts of health and wellbeing that are being promulgated through those marketing campaigns. Lastly, it asks what kinds of impact fast-moving nutraceuticals are likely to have on the lives of India's rural poor. It concludes by questioning how smooth a transition to nutraceutical consumption Big Food marketing strategies can really achieve and how readily low-income families seeking to feed their families and safeguard health will actually adopt concepts of wellness and internalise micro-nutrient associated risks.

What are nutraceuticals?

The US physician, Dr Stephen De Felice, claims to have coined the term 'nutraceuticals' in 1989 as follows: 'A food or part of a food that provides medical or health benefits, including the prevention and/or treatment of a disease'. For De Felice, this category includes any food that we already eat, but which molecular and clinical research establishes as having a particular health benefit. In other words, according to this definition, a food can become a nutraceutical simply through the production of new scientific knowledge. As food science has developed in relation to advances in molecular biology, the term has more commonly come to refer to foods that have been transformed and enhanced through technological processes to have particular health-giving properties. Such processes include the fortification of foods with vitamins and minerals, the biofortification of food through plant breeding for nutrient-rich crops and the manufacture of dietary supplements.

Despite the wide circulation of the term and its inclusion in the Oxford English Dictionary, a review of the literature shows that nutraceuticals do not yet constitute a legal entity or specific object of regulation in any country. Instead, the term has largely been used and promoted by representatives from the global food industry, for whom the nutraceutical's association with scientific evidence and medicine generates additional economic value. Indeed, nutraceuticals might be defined as food products that have been created solely for the capacity to make health claims about them (Katan & Roos, 2004; Schneider, n.d.).

How did the privately manufactured and marketed nutraceutical product also become a cornerstone of the global development agenda? By the late 1990s, international development organisations such as UNICEF or the World Bank, had shifted from talking about hunger as a function of poverty and famine to talking about 'hidden hunger'. The focus was now on the quality as well as the quantity of food, and the qualities that foods have were monitored at a molecular level. Hidden hunger was defined as a lack of micronutrients – vitamins and minerals such as iron, zinc, vitamin A and iodine. As the food sociologist Kimura notes, over the course of the 1990s, the hidden hunger concept slowly accrued global authority through discussion at a series of international conferences on nutrition, global food security and child health, including the 1990 World Summit for Children, the 1991 Montreal meeting 'ending hidden hunger', the 1992 International Conference on Nutrition and the 1996 World Food Summit (Kimura, 2008). The global consensus that micronutrient deficiency is a high priority area is today indicated by its incorporation into the programs of bi-lateral and multi-lateral development agencies such as DFID and AUSAID and its inclusion in the first Millennium Development Goal.[2]

The global distribution of micronutrient deficiency is now monitored, measured and mapped by a growing number of international organisations and academics.[3] By all these measures, India's rates of hidden hunger are alarmingly high. India alone boasts the world's largest undernourished population – over 200 million. Fifty-six percent of ever-married women and 70% of children under the age of five are anemic (International Institute for Population Science (IIPS) and Macro International, 2007) and at least 15% are at risk of iodine deficiency (Chakravarty & Sinha, 2002). In this context, the affordable nutraceutical that is designed for the rural poor is celebrated as a humanitarian technology, capable of relieving suffering and ameliorating the loss of life in contexts of crisis (Cross, 2013; Redfield, 2012).

The notion of hidden hunger has also been picked up by the international economic community, who draw on medical research about the effects of micronutrient deficiency on long-term health and mental development to make links between hidden hunger and human capital. It is the shift from 'general' improvements in health to the specified mental and physical benefits of micronutrients that has been significant for economists at institutions like Asian Development Bank (ADB, 2004) and World Bank (2006): well-nourished people, it is claimed, are able to 'work harder and be potentially more innovative …' (Bekefi, 2006, p. 8). The link between micronutrient deficiency and economic development is rendered concrete and measured by disability-adjusted life years (DALYs), with a recent study suggesting that India lost 1000 DALYs to micronutrient deficiencies per 100,000 population (Muthayya et al., 2013, p. 8). Based partly on DALY estimates, the Copenhagen Consensus of 2004 convened by a panel of distinguished economists determined that after the control of HIV/AIDS, providing micronutrients had the best economic benefit-to-cost ratio of alleviating poverty in the developing world (Copenhagen Consensus Center, 2004).

The notion of deficiency in vitamins or minerals is not new. Governments have been providing vitamin and iron supplements, for example, to pregnant women since the 1970s. However, the growing prominence of the concept of 'micronutrients' as a scientific category and the concept of 'hidden hunger' as a major cause of ill-health and poverty in the development industry has coincided with, on the one hand, developments in food science that have enabled the isolation and transformation of individual bioactive components in foods (Kim, 2012, p. 7) and on the other hand, the growing consensus that food fortification is the best solution to micronutrient deficiency.

Like its counterpart, obesity, micronutrient deficiency has been 'artifactually constructed' through epidemiological measures and economic algorithms in ways that shape its problematisation and subsequent interventions (Guthman, 2013). Since the 1990s, we have seen the demise of alternative solutions to micronutrient deficiency, such as supplementation, kitchen gardens or dietary education, in favour of the notion that the most effective and efficient point of transformation for established diets is the corporate laboratory (Morris, Cogill, & Uauy, 2008; Victora, 2009, p. 1124). As a World Bank report describes food fortification: 'Probably no other technology available today offers as large an opportunity to improve lives and accelerate development at such low cost and in such a short time' (The World Bank, 1994). Affordable fortified foods have emerged as the site of opportunity in which market growth, healthy economies and humanitarian ethics coincide.

Public-private partnership

With the shift from poverty and hunger to hidden hunger and micronutrient deficiency, government responses to malnutrition have expanded from direct humanitarian action through food aid to the creation of an 'enabling environment', in which affordable fortified food markets can flourish. In India, the Integrated Child Development Scheme began in 1975 as a subsidised food program that distributes basic foods such as wheat and grain to poor families in *anganwadi* centres, village-level centres for government-funded social welfare programmes. Yet, 30 years after the establishment of the ICDS, the most recent National Family Health Survey reported that 48% of the country's children under 5 are stunted, 20% are wasted and 43% are underweight (International Institute for Population Science (IIPS) and Macro International, 2007). The state-sponsored food program has been widely criticised for its inefficiency and corruption. More recently, the influential development economists Abhijit Banerjee and Esther Duflo have argued that food subsidies, which are designed to ameliorate poverty-related hunger, are an inadequate response to micronutrient deficiency because they fail to address the fact that the poor can usually afford to buy enough food but *prioritise* better-tasting food:

> Developing ways to pack foods that people like to eat with additional nutrients, and coming up with new strains of nutritious and tasty crops that can be grown in a wider range of environments, need to become priorities for food technology, on an equal footing with raising productivity. (Banerjee & Duflo, 2011, 40)

Packing better-tasting food with micronutrients is where the private sector is seen to have skills and resources that are not always available to governments. While the state is still thought to have a role in regulation and facilitation, the private sector is increasingly considered to have the intellectual property, manufacturing capacities and marketing skills needed to take food fortification the last mile (Kimura, 2013). Public–private partnership is now the favoured model for improving nutrition in developing countries for the World Bank, the WHO and the Millennium Project taskforce on Hunger.

In 2002, the UN established the Global Alliance for Improved Nutrition (GAIN) as a collaborative mechanism for business, civil society and governmental organisations to address micronutrient challenges worldwide. GAIN received funding from the Bill and Melinda Gates Foundation, the Canadian Development Agency, USAID and administrative support from the UNDP. It provides funding for public–private national fortification programs, for research to remove technical challenges in food fortification and to support market mechanisms for securing access to fortified foods. To obtain a GAIN grant, the organisation requires that each country establish a National Fortification Alliance, made up of government and corporate membership, to ensure that the appropriate foods are fortified and that they are made available through market mechanisms. GAIN aims to provide corporations with technical assistance to scale up access to their products through facilitating partnerships such as school feeding programs, joint awareness-raising and educational activities with organisations such as UNICEF and the Flour Fortification Initiative, assistance in social marketing and helping to promote food fortification through publications and reports. In 2008, GAIN opened an India office to assist NGOs and businesses to create and distribute 'market viable' fortified foods to the rural population.

With funding from GAIN and the World Bank Institute, the Business Alliance for Food Fortification was launched in Beijing 2005 to promote relationships between the food industry and the international development sector. The BAFF's purpose, as stated on their website, is to 'identify new financial mechanisms and new business models, expand scientific knowledge and expertise in fortification, and catalyse joint action between companies, development partners, and government'. The private sector, it states, is crucial in providing the products, technology and marketing for the creation of 'market-viable and sustainable food fortification'. For multinational companies like Coca-Cola or Unilever, who are co-chairs of the BAFF, or Danone, who joined the GAIN board in 2006, these organisations create opportunities for collaboration and networking with representatives from government and development agencies, and access to public and philanthropic funding and political support. All these companies are seeking to expand their fortified foods portfolios in India.

Today, Coca-Cola, PepsiCo and GlaxoSmithKline each distribute and market their bottom-of-the-pyramid nutraceutical products in partnership with local NGOs and microenterprise organisations. In many cases, these NGOs have received funding from global organisations like UNICEF; in some cases, mediated by GAIN, to provide educational programs on micronutrients in rural areas. Educational campaigns by NGOs and development agencies that are run in concert with the rollout of new fortified food products prime a market for corporate access. Such partnerships are indications of the 'creeping privatisation of health education' (Powell, 2014). For their Nutristar™ drink fortified with patented triple-fortification technology for iron, vitamin A and iodine, for example, Proctor & Gamble partnered with UNICEF, who provided health education about micronutrients, at the same time as Proctor & Gamble distributed the product.

These partnerships have also been crucial to 'last-mile' distribution strategies. In Orissa, Coca-Cola partnered with the NGO BISWA to distribute Vitingo™ through self help groups; in Andhra Pradesh, GlaxoSmithKline developed a partnership with SKS Microfinance, a microcredit organisation, to distribute Asha™. The distribution of nutraceutical products in rural areas is being tied into direct-selling employment opportunities, with rural distributors being both personal consumers of the product and social conduits through whom companies can access wider social networks (Cross & Street, 2009). When GlaxosmithKline launched Asha™, it added 4000 sub-distributors to its existing 500 distributors in small towns (Kashyap & Raut, 2008, p. 552).

To its champions, this partnership model for affordable nutraceuticals is celebrated as a mechanism for enabling access to vital health products and an engine of entrepreneurship and rural employment (Dolan, Johnstone-Louis, & Scott, 2012). Yet, its critics have highlighted the ways in which GAIN's support for multinational companies crowd out local businesses, leading to the loss of local industry and employment opportunities. Meanwhile, nutritionists have raised questions about the nutritional quality of fortified foods that are also laced with sugar and salt i.e. where 'better tasting' also corresponds with being damaging to health (see Nestle, 2013) and social activists have queried the potentially dangerous marketing activities of GAIN partners such as Nestle, in relation to infant feeding and complementary foods for young children. In a decision that appears to suggest such concerns are taken seriously, in January 2013, the WHO decided to postpone formal relations with GAIN on the basis of its links to the food industry and the need for further information on its partners' compliance with WHO nutritional policy (WHO, 2013).

Harnessing science

Key to the added value that fortification lends food is its scientific evidence base. This is also where multinational corporations have a distinct advantage over local competitors. The acquisition of nutraceutical portfolios has become increasingly attractive to corporations already invested in pharmaceuticals, such as GlaxoSmithKline. According to market analysts, pharmaceuticals have increasingly narrow profit margins, especially in developing world contexts where generics are providing greater competition (e.g. Frost & Sullivan, 2011). Over the past three years, following consultant advice, GlaxoSmithKline has begun to shed its pharmaceutical portfolio and expand its nutra-ceutical portfolio in the BRIC economies. Nutraceuticals have lower profit margins than pharmaceuticals but require a fraction of the outlay on research and development (IKON Marketing Consultants, 2013). At the same time, nutraceuticals are seen as an opportunity for India's food industry and fast-moving consumer goods industry to increase revenues. Making claims about the health-giving qualities of particular prod-ucts enables multi-nationals to sell more expensive products in a highly competitive, often locally dominated, marketplace (Bourne Partners, 2013). In a widely circulated newsletter, the accountancy firm Price Waterhouse Coopers (PWC) recently identified increased collaboration between the fast-moving consumer goods(FMCG) sector and the pharmaceutical industry as the primary opportunity for innovation in the nutraceuticals sector (PWC, 2013).

A clear sign of the pharmaceuticalisation of food is the establishment of scientific foundations and institutes by food and FMCG companies in India to generate the scien-tific evidence needed to market their products as nutraceuticals. For example, Coca-Cola established the Beverage Institute for Health & Wellness in 2004; Brittania established the Brittania Nutritional Foundation in 2009; and GlaxoSmithKline launched the Horlicks Nutrition Academy in 2011. These institutes conduct research to establish micronutrient deficiency in target populations and on the products developed to meet that deficiency. One effect of corporate-funded scientific research into micronutrient deficiency is that homemade food and established diets are considered inadequate and in need of fortification with commercial foods that can be better quantified and moni-tored in terms of their micronutrient content. As Kimura argues, 'nutritionism' – the reduction of food to its nutritional qualities – has shifted authority over food production and consumption from a domestic to scientific domain (Kimura, 2013). The Horlicks Nutrition Academy website, for example, features photographs of scientists in white coats and emphasises their expertise in nutritional science: 'Our panel of scientists, nutritionists and researchers are committed to provide you with the expertise and nutri-tional solutions to help you lead a healthier life'.[4] Indeed, Kimura argues that fortified baby food is attractive to policy-makers precisely because of its 'potential to bypass mothers as the gatekeeper of babies' health' (Kimura, 2008, p. 234). Being a responsi-ble mother in developing countries now entails 'choosing' food products that have undergone corporate fortification (ibid., p. 251).

GAIN actively encourages governments to endorse products that make scientifically valid claims. And yet, as critics have pointed out, most of the scientific evidence for the efficacy of nutraceuticals is generated by the corporations themselves. Indeed, there is almost no regulation of the effectiveness and quality of nutraceuticals in India, pre-cisely because they do not occupy a distinct legal category from food and beverages. It is therefore much easier to make health claims about fortified foods in India than drugs.

In making scientific claims, the nutraceutical industry has borrowed from the pharmaceutical industry its dominant product testing mechanism: the randomised con-trolled trial. The results of randomised controlled trials are converted into DALYs, which enable corporations to scale up the 'cost-effectiveness' of nutraceutical products to a national level. As critics have pointed out, however, randomised controlled trials take place in highly controlled environments and tell us little about the impact of nutraceuticals in places where compliance may not be high:

The types of delivery systems used, country characteristics, year in which the study was done, program characteristics, and costing methodologies contribute to the variability in cost estimates found in the literature. It is not clear whether these cost estimates include expenses necessary to attain such high compliance rates. (Berry, Mukherjee, & Shastry, 2012, p. 6)

What corporate-funded nutritional academies research and how, what is left out of those studies (e.g. the effects of poor nutritional content, such as sugar and salt, or the local availability of nutritional foods) and how evidence from those studies is subsequently drawn on to market corporate products or garner political support demand enquiry from social scientists equivalent to recent research on the politics of evidence in the pharmaceutical industry (McGoey, 2012; Will & Moreira, 2010).

Selling wellness

How do you make a nutraceutical market for the rural poor? As the rising costs of health care put it beyond reach of much of this population, investment analysts anticipate that they will become increasingly susceptible to notions of wellness and its associated products. And yet the cornerstone of 'wellness', the micronutrient, is not a familiar concept for much of the Indian population: 'The Indian consumer's awareness about conventional nutraceutical ingredients such as omega-3 fatty acids or lutein is severely limited, and nutraceutical manufacturers need to take up the cause and spread awareness about their products to the Indian masses' (Frost & Sullivan, 2011, p. 5). The major challenge in this area is considered to be that of translating the established acceptance of alternative and herbal remedies and supplements in Indian ayurveda traditions into concepts of 'wellness' and 'micro-nutrient deficiency'. The problem is how to make people think about their food and their bodies in terms of micronutrient content and the long-term health risks associated with micronutrient deficiency.

One of the reasons why Horlicks, and the fortified beverage market in general, does so well in India may be because the commodification of ayurveda tonics is already well established. Companies like Himalayan, for example, repackage ayurveda herbal preparations 'in the symbolic forms of biomedical, "English", medicine – brightly coloured capsules, plastic bottles, English labels – and [distribute] it by prescription through biomedical physicians' (Cohen, 2000, p. 133). Indeed, companies like Horlicks achieve many of their sales through the prescription of their products by family physicians. As one marketing analyst report put it: 'The existence of alternative medicine in India, and the Indian consumer's belief in them, could provide a platform for the nutraceutical industry to capitalize on' (Frost & Sullivan, 2011, p. 5).

Recent research on nutraceuticals in medical anthropology and sociology has concentrated on the ways in which the transformation of food into a micronutrient health product transforms people's sense of self and their relationship to their body in ways that afford new techniques of health governance (Herrick, 2011; Powell, 2014). It is suggested that the introduction of nutraceuticals is associated with a growing concern with the 'risks' of living (Kim, 2012) and the fostering of individual responsibility for managing the risk of chronic disease. Food becomes another everyday space in which we monitor our health status and 'a molecular understanding of foods … expands into the social realm' (ibid., p. 12; Rose, 2007).

The majority of this research, however, has been carried out in urban, middle class environments, often in middle- or high-income countries. As a consequence, there remains little understanding of the concepts of 'wellness' that may be emerging in the context of nutraceutical products designed as humanitarian technologies for the rural poor. In rural India, corporations recognise the need to market their affordable products through associations with different aspirational teleologies from those they use to market products to urban consumers. Where the standard Horlicks is marketed on the basis of people's aspirations for their children's educational achievement and the prevention of future 'lifestyle' diseases, for example, affordable Horlicks was rebranded as 'Asha™', meaning hope. This was partly to avoid contamination of the Horlicks brand with 'poor' associations, but it also suggests that marketing agencies believe consumption in rural families, where poor health and hunger may already be the norm, is not oriented towards the prevention of ill-health, but rather a future where the health and prospects of their children may improve. The product sells the possibility for survival amidst the struggle to sustain life in the present.

Established supplementary food practices in rural India are seen by the nutraceutical industry as an opportunity to sell fortified foods. But how easily can one set of foods and practices be metaphorically extended to incorporate another? As education and marketing campaigns are rolled out alongside nutraceutical products, will women in rural Andhra Pradesh and Orissa internalise a notion of the molecular self? Will they see commercially produced nutraceuticals as better, more scientifically valid versions of the everyday foods that they give their children to promote vitality and growth? Or will nutraceuticals be received as overly expensive foods? The possibility that food marketing experiments, such as those of micropackaging or direct selling, that are explicitly designed to overcome obstacles associated with frontier markets in culturally unfamiliar and logistically difficult environments may be less successful than anticipated is suggested by the disappearance of Asha™ from the GlaxoSmithKline website and the absence of any publicly available information on the product since its test marketing stage in 2010.

The hegemonic power exerted by multinational food companies through integrated marketing techniques used to promote unhealthy foods is well documented (e.g. Jackson, Harrison, Swinburn, & Lawrence, 2014). How successful rural marketing techniques such as multilevel marketing are in promoting new concepts of health and wellness is, by comparison, relatively underexplored. This is where future in-depth, ethnographic research capable of detailing the rich worlds of food and health practices into which multinational companies seek entry for their nutraceutical products will be crucial.

Conclusion

On the one hand, new partnerships between international development organisations and the food industry and new strategies for accessing nutraceutical markets at 'the bottom of the pyramid' need to be approached critically. The increasingly dominant message that commercially fortified foods are the solution to hidden hunger obviates the importance of living conditions and structural impediments that may prevent families from creating a balanced diet. Indeed, we should be asking why fortified foods have replaced a balanced diet as the basis for nutritional health and what is at stake in such transitions when they are made in the name of humanitarianism. As the nutritionist Marion Nestle pointed out in 2002, 'The complexity of food composition means that no single nutrient is likely to work nearly so well as a diet rich in the fruits and vegetables from which that nutrient was isolated' (Nestle, 2013 [2002], Part Five).

On the other hand, it is important to bear in mind the logistical, economic and cultural limitations that multinational food companies face when they seek to make new markets for nutraceutical products. It is tempting to emphasise the 'smooth' segue of corporate capitalism into the world of humanitarian food (Errington, Fujikura, & Gewertz, 2012). But the amalgamation of the values of profit and humanitarianism in a single nutraceutical product is an achievement that must be actively and repeatedly brokered in the conference halls of the international development sector, the reports of marketing consultants and analysts, the pot-holed roads of India's rural districts and the homes of rural distributors and Indian consumers. As research on analogous products, such as the selling of soap (Cross & Street, 2009) or solar lanterns (Cross, 2013) as public health goods has indicated, multinationals often encounter rougher social and physical terrain in rural markets than they anticipate. Just how far the nutraceutical can travel remains an important question for capitalists, development specialists, consumers and social scientists alike.

Acknowledgement

A version of this paper was first presented at the University of Sussex Pharmaceuticals and Global Health conference in June 2013. I am grateful to two anonymous reviewers and to Jamie Cross for their helpful comments.

Funding

This research was supported by funding from the Nuffield Foundation under [grant number NCF/36321] and the Economic and Social Research Foundation under [grant number Es/L003147/1].

Notes

1. Fast-moving consumer goods refer to products sold quickly, at a low cost and often in a small unit size.
2. Despite the apparent shift from quantity to quality, USAID's food programs have recently been attacked by Medecins Sans Frontieres on precisely the basis that the agricultural surplus they are offloading onto poor countries through their food aid program fails to meet the United States' own nutritional standards. See http://www.msf.org/article/open-letter-us-government-about-quality-food-aid.
3. See, for example, the World Health Organisation (WHO) database on anaemia http://www.who.int/vmnis/database/anaemia/en/; the wiki map of iron deficiency adjusted DALY's using data from WHO, http://commons.wikimedia.org/wiki/File:Iron-deficiency_anaemia_world_map_-_DALY_-_WHO2002.svg; The World Bank's regional table of DALYs lost by attributing to nutritional deficiencies (Caulfield, Richard, Rivera, Musgrove, & Black, 2006) and the micronutrient initiative's overview of data limitations http://www.micronutrient.org/resources/publications/mn_report.pdf; and most recently, the creation of a hidden hunger index and its mapping in relation to DALY's (Muthayya et al., 2013).
4. http://www.horlicksnutritionacademy.com/AboutHNA.aspx.

References

Asian Development Bank. (2004). *Food fortification in Asia: Improving health and building economies* (ADB Nutrition and Development Series No. 7). Manila: Author.

Banerjee, A., & Duflo, E. (2011). *Poor economics: A radical rethinking of the way to fight global poverty.* New York, NY: Public Affairs.

Bekefi, T. (2006). *Business as a partner in tackling micronutrient deficiency: Lessons in multisectoral partnership* (Corporate Social Responsibility Initiative Report). John F. Kennedy School of Government, Harvard University. Retrieved from http://www.hks.harvard.edu/m-rcbg/CSRI/publications/report_7_Bekefi_micronutrient_2006FNL1-23-07.pdf

Berry, J., Mukherjee, P., & Shastry, G. K. (2012). Taken with a grain of salt? Micronutrient fortification in South Asia *CESifo Economic Studies, 58*, 422–449.

Bourne Partners. (2013). *Sector report: Nutraceuticals industry.* Charlotte, NC: Author.

Caulfield, L. E., Richard, S. A., Rivera, J. A., Musgrove, P., & Black, R. E. (2006). Stunting, wasting, and micronutrient deficiency disorders. In D. T. Jamison & J. G. Breman (Eds.), *Disease control priorities in developing countries* (2nd ed., pp. 551–567). Washington, DC: World Bank.

Chakravarty, I., & Sinha, R. (2002). Prevalence of micronutrient deficiency based on obtained from the national pilot program of micronutrient malnutrition results on control. *Nutrition Reviews, 60*, 53–58.

Cohen, L. (2000). *No aging in India: Alzheimer's, the bad family, and other modern things.* Berkeley: University of California Press.

Copenhagen Consensus Center. (2004). *The results of Copenhagen Consensus 2004.* Retrieved from http://www.copenhagenconsensus.com/Default.aspx?ID=699

Cross, J. (2013). The 100th object: Solar lighting technology and humanitarian goods. *Journal of Material Culture, 18*, 367–387.

Cross, J., & Street, A. (2009). Anthropology at the bottom of the pyramid. *Anthropology Today, 25*, 4–9.

Dolan, C., Johnstone-Louis, M., & Scott, L. (2012). Shampoo, saris and SIM cards: Seeking entrepreneurial futures at the bottom of the pyramid. *Gender & Development, 20*, 33–47.

Ernst & Young. (2012). *Nutraceuticals: A critical supplement for building a healthy India.* New Delhi: FICCI.

Errington, F., Fujikura, T., & Gewertz, D. (2012). Instant noodles as an antifriction device: Making the BOP with PPP in PNG. *American Anthropologist, 114*, 19–31.

Frost & Sullivan. (2011). *Global nutraceuticals industry: Investing in healthy living.* Mumbai: Author.

Gupta, A. (2009, March 8). Special report: Health, wellness and more. *Business India*, 61–64.

Guthman, J. (2013). Fatuous measures: The artifactual construction of the obesity epidemic. *Critical Public Health, 23*, 263–273.

Herrick, C. (2011). *Governing health and consumption: Sensible citizens, behaviour and the city.* Bristol: Policy Press.

Ikon Marketing Consultants. (2013). *The Indian nutraceuticals market: Poised from neutral to top gear.* Ahmedabad: IKON.

Indian Business News Agency. (2012). *Indian nutraceuticals market forecast to 2017.* New Delhi: IBNA.

International Institute for Population Science (IIPS) and Macro International. (2007). *National Family Health Survey (NFHS-3), 2005–6.* Mumbai: IIPS.

Jackson, M., Harrison, P., Swinburn, B., & Lawrence, M. (2014). Unhealthy food, integrated marketing communication and power: A critical analysis. *Critical Public Health, 24*, 489–505.

Kashyap, P., & Raut, S. (2008). *The rural marketing book (text & practice).* Pondicherry: Dorling Kindersley India.

Katan, M., & Roos, N. (2004). Promises and problems of functional foods. *Critical Reviews in Food Science and Nutrition, 44*, 369–377.

Kim, H. (2012). Functional foods and the biomedicalisation of everyday life: A case of germinated brown rice. *Sociology of Health & Illness, 35*, 842–857.

Kimura, A. H. (2008). Who defines babies' 'Needs'?: The scientization of baby food in Indonesia. *Social Politics: International Studies in Gender, State & Society, 15*, 232–260.

Kimura, A. H. (2013). *Hidden hunger: Gender and the politics of smarter foods.* Ithaca: Cornell University Press.

McGoey, L. (2012). The logic of strategic ignorance. *The British Journal of Sociology, 63*, 533–576.

Morris, S. S., Cogill, B., & Uauy, R. (2008). Effective international action against undernutrition: Why has it proven so difficult and what can be done to accelerate progress? *The Lancet, 371*, 608–621.

Muthayya, S., Rah, J. H., Sugimoto, J. D., Roos, F. F., Kraemer, K., & Black, R. E. (2013). The global hidden hunger indices and maps: An advocacy tool for action. *PLoS One, 8*, e67860.

Nestle, M. (2013). *Food politics: How the food industry influences nutrition and health.* Berkeley, CA: University California Press. Ebook.

Powell, D. (2014). Childhood obesity, corporate philanthropy and the creeping privatisation of health education. *Critical Public Health, 24*, 226–238.

Prahalad, C. K. (2009). *The fortune at the bottom of the pyramid: Eradicating poverty through profits.* London: Prentice Hall.

Price Waterhouse Coopers. (2013, March). Food as pharma: As wellness products evolve, the distinction between food and medicine blurs. *R & C Worlds Express.* Retrieved from http://www.pwc.com/r&c

Redfield, P. (2012). Bioexpectations: Life technologies as humanitarian goods. *Public Culture, 24*, 157–184.

Rose, N. (2007). *The politics of life itself.* Princeton, NJ: Princeton University Press.

Schneider, T. (n.d.). *Functional foods: Are they sociologically interesting?* Conference paper presented at the TASA Conference, University of Tasmania, 6–8 December 2005.

Techsi Research. (2013). *Indian nutraceuticals market forecast and opportunities, 2017.* Noida: Author.

The World Bank. (1994). *Enriching lives: Overcoming vitamin and mineral malnutrition in developing countries.* Washington, DC: Author.

The World Bank. (2006). *Repositioning Nutrition as central to the development agenda: A strategy for large-scale action.* Washington, DC: Author.

Victora, C. G. (2009). Nutrition in early life: A global priority. *The Lancet, 374*, 1123–1125.

Will, C., & Moreira, T. (2010). *Medical proofs, social experiments: Clinical trials in shifting contexts.* Farnham: Ashgate.

World Health Organisation. (2013). *Document EB132.R9: Relations with nongovernmental organisations.* Retrieved from http://apps.who.int/gb/ebwha/pdf_files/EB132/B132_R9-en.pdf

Index

Abrams, Martin 124
Access to Nutrition Index (ATNI) 75, 90
Advertising Standards Authority (ASA) (New Zealand) 87
Africa: cereals 7; maize 6; meat 6, 17; poultry 6; soft drinks 67 *see also* Kenya, case study on
agriculture 18, 25–9, 31, 63
alcohol 43
American Beverage Association (ABA) 64, 109, 112–13
Asia: Central Asia 6; meat 6, 9, 17; nutrition transition/Big Food diet 55; palm oil 6, 17; pig meat 9; South East Asia 6, 17; soybean oil 6; sugar/sweeteners 9 *see also* China; India
Asian Development Bank (ADB) 139
Aujan Industries 67
Australia: children, marketing 50, 81–2, 87; core food products 42; Healthy Australia Commitment (AFGC) 89; outdoor advertising 37; public policies and commitments of multinationals 2, 77–91; schools, advertising in vicinity of 50
Australian Association of National Advertisers (AANA) 87
Australian Beverages Council (ABC) 87, 89
Australian Food and Grocery Council (AFGC): Quick Service Restaurant Initiative for Responsible Advertising and Marketing to Children (QSR) 81, 87; Responsible Children Marketing Initiative (RCMI) 81–2, 87
Austin, J Paul 61

baby food, fortification of 142
Banerjee, Abhijit 140
banner advertising on websites 99, 102
Barnoya, J 49
barriers to market entry 56, 60–2
Barrios, Art 117
Bates, Nat 113
Better-for-You Portfolio (PepsiCo) 124

'better for you' products 1, 2, 98–9, 125, 129, 131
Beverage Institute for Health & Wellness (BIHW) 142
beverages: alcohol 43; atoles 49; cereals, marketing of 95; economic development 13–18; fortification 136–7, 143; Guatemala 48–51; India 136–7, 141, 143–4; Kenya 29; Mongolia 37–45; Philippines 37–45; schools, advertising in vicinity of 37–45, 48–51 *see also* soft drinks industry
Biden, Joe 62
Big Food diet *see* nutrition transition/Big Food diet
BISWA 141
Blumenthal, Richard 101
bottled water 41, 49, 58–9, 66, 137
Bragg, MA 51
brands: cereals, marketing of 96, 99, 101–3, 128; characters 99; China 56, 62; equity 62; exposure 50–1; funness 128–30; Guatemala, snack food advertising in vicinity of schools in 47, 50–1; India 56, 62, 67, 136, 144; loyalty 23; messages 37; policies and commitments of multinationals 78–9, 81; schools, marketing in vicinity of 38-40, 42–3, 50–1
Britannia Nutritional Foundation 142
Brownell, Kelly D 56–7, 63–7, 104
Bryson, John 62
Business Alliance for Food Fortification (BAFF) 140–1

California *see* soda tax initiatives in California, media coverage of
California Center for Public Health Advocacy 116
Canada 14, 48, 127–8
cancer 31, 75, 77, 108, 137
capture of political agencies by industry 56, 63
cardiovascular disease/heart disease 4, 17, 95, 109, 137
Carter, Jimmy 61

Milton Keynes UK
Ingram Content Group UK Ltd.
UKHW051925141024
449569UK00027B/1369